Angelo Barbato

ZERO DESEASE

Original title: **Malattia zero**
Translated by: **Clarissa Cassels**

Publisher: **Tektime**

ZERO DISEASE

The birth of the health collaborative model (Commons).

The birth of digital networks for health (Health Smart Grid Digital).

Author: Angelo Barbato MD angelo.barbato@gmail.com

Doctor of Hygiene and Preventive Medicine Specialist and Specializing in Cardiology. Expert in Public and Private Health. He has worked in the Health Management of Italian health organizations, military and civil covering clinical positions, Chief of Health Director of Public Hospital, Chief of Health Director in Local Health Authority, Chief of DATA Management and Chief of ICT Management. He is coordinator of the Technical Board "Disease Zero and Sustainable Health" of CETRI-TIRES Third Industrial Revolution European Society, inspired by the economic ideas of Jeremy Rifkin.

Index

Index

Presentation

The book stems from the desire of the authors to disseminate tools and transformation of models in health care, inspired
by Jeremy Rifkin's theory 'Zero Marginal Cost'.

The ambitious attempt to make an accessible and usable
participative model of health, illness and treatment, meets the
need of the human being to recover the relationship with himself
and with the world around him. The environmental, economic,
social and technological should be geared towards preserving the
human being and the environment he lives in. The inevitable
repercussions on health will become increasingly avoidable using
the new paradigm of communication, through conscientious
choices and the essential support of the internet. The transition
from a Hierarchical and Structured Medicine to a Capillary and
Distributed one sees the human being involved in the role of being responsible for himself. The health-oriented community will
be the arrival point, not only a start, and a social duty prior to being a fundamental right.

This probably represents a visionary shift which, in the
words of our intellectual reference "It's Already Happening".

Contributions

Thank you to the following professionals for their contribution:

→ **Bruno Corda, MD**
Doctor, Specialized in Emergency and First Aid Surgery, Hygiene and Preventive Medicine. Already a Family Doctor, Director of Prevention Department, Director of Public Hygiene and Health Service. President of the Italian Society of Hygiene- Lazio Section. Master Degree CORGESAN and EMMAS in Health Management. Technical Table "Zero Disease and Sustainable Health" of CETRI-TIRES - Third Industrial Revolution European Society, inspired by the economic ideas of Jeremy Rifkin. bruno_corda@alice.it

A special thanks to Bruno Corda for having introduced me to the studies of Jeremy Rifkin.

Angelo Barbato

→ **Angela Meggiolaro, MD**
Specialized Doctor in the Department of Hygiene and Infectious Disease Department of Sapienza, University of Rome. Epidemiologic and Health Economy Field experience. Author of textbooks and Scientific Publications in the Field of Public Health and Medicine of the Territory. Technical Table "Zero Disease and Sustainable Health" of CETRI-TIRES - Third Industrial Revolution European Society, inspired by the economic ideas of Jeremy Rifkin. angela.meggiolaro@gmail.com

→ **Dr. Angelo Consoli**
Director of the European Office of Jeremy Rifkin
President of CETRI-TIRES (Third Industrial Revolution Euro-

pean Society)
Co-Author with Livio de Santoli of the Manifesto-book "Zero Zone".

→ **Francesca Mirabelli, MD Ph.D**
Specialist in Cardiology
Ph.D in Biomedical technology in clinical medicine
Second level Master Degree in Imaging diagnostic   cardiology
ASL Rome 1. francesca.mirabelli78@gmail.com

→ **Alessandro Anselmo, MD Ph.D**
Specialist in General Surgery
Ph.D in Surgical pathophysiology
Ph.D in Organ Transplants
Second level Master Degree in Organ Transplants
Fellow of the European Board of Surgery
Medical Executive - UOC Transplant Surgery - PTV Foundation- Rome

→ **Antonio Magi, MD**
  Doctor Specialist in Radiology
  Health Past-Director IV District ASL Rome A

→ **Dr. Roberto Del Gaudio**
  Personal Trainer Master 3° level federal FIPE CONI and Jurist
  roberto.del.gaudio2@gmail.com

→ **Dr. Antonina Fazio**
  Biologist-Nutritionist Specialized in Clinical Pathology
  afazio2002@hotmail.com

→ **Dr. Eloisa Fioravanti**
  Degree in Arts and Dentistry fioravelo@gmail.com

Translated by Clarissa A. Cassels
Degree in European Studies at Maastricht University
Translator and interpreter, massage therapist and travel blogger on www.piglinaround.com

Foreword by Angelo Consoli – The Health Communities

The **Third Industrial Revolution** is not only a change from a centralized, top-down energy/economic model towards a distributive and interactive one.

The Third Industrial Revolution is also and mostly a **paradigmatic** shift for the human race.

An epical passage from an individualistic and utilitarian lifestyle to a biospheric and empathic one. In a society in which the marginal cost of production and distribution of goods and services is closer and closer to zero, where information, objects, ideas, services and people travel at infinitesimal costs compared to a hundred years ago, and in timeframes then unimaginable; the human genre is emerging from an economy of scarcity, entering a sustainable system of abundance. An economy in which its activity will no longer develop according to the canons and standards of the traditional market economy based on profit, but according to canons and standards of a social economy based on **collaborative Commons.**

Jeremy Rifkin lucidly describes **Energy** Commons as composed of millions of prosumers (both producers and consumers) able to generate almost all their green energy needs at a marginal cost close to nothing , the Commons of **Logistics** able to project, print and distribute goods and services at almost null marginal costs, and the Commons of Health, Education and Culture able to guarantee scholastic, health and cultural services of same condition; or Mobility Commons for the movement of humans in increasingly sustainable, efficient and economic ways.

The new generations are projected beyond the capitalist market and the centralized, hierarchical, closed, patriarchal, property-tied model towards a **distributed model**, which is collaborative, open, transparent, equal and empathic.

It is what Rifkin calls power on a lateral scale, or "**Lateral Power**".

Today's youth, linked together in a virtual sphere (by social networks through which information travels with abundance and freely) and in a physical space (thanks to low cost flights, unimaginable ten years ago, or faster and more efficient metropolitan transport lines), "are rapidly getting rid of the remaining ideological cultural and commercial ties that have long been separating the "mine" from the "yours", in the frame of a capitalistic system characterized by relationships of private property, market exchanges and national borders. "**Open Source**" has become the mantra of a generation that sees power relations in a completely new way compared to their parents and grandparents who have lived in a world dominated by geopolitics." (cit. Jeremy Rifkin, Society at Zero Marginal Cost, pag. 429-430)

In a new empathic civilization profoundly integrated in the biosphere community, all our natural resources will become **shared patrimony** and the way that they are used will become everyone's business.Even the planning of urban spaces, be it industrial or rural, will not be an exception to this rule.

The construction of large industrial and infrastructure installation networks of the third millennium and the third industrial revolution cannot therefore continue to proceed according to the dissipative and unsustainable canons of the fossil era. Networks **were built in disregard** of the principles of efficiency, space optimization of urban and rural spaces were ravaged repeatedly and savagely for the construction of tens of thousands of power lines, pipelines, cable ducts, aqueducts, road infrastructure, electronic networks and lighting networks.

In the collaborative Commons idea, the **internet of things** offers new and unreleased possibilities of "doing more with less" (the principle of energetic efficiency affirmed by the European Union) taking advantage of the existing networks and enriching them with new functions, useful to expand the **sharing economy** and **empathy** among human beings.

The collaborative Commons is based on the idea that the **thermodynamic laws** cannot be ignored, minimized, avoided or violated. The **first law of thermodynamics** clearly tells us that nothing is destroyed but everything is transformed. Therefore, burning an object to close the waste cycle does not at all entail its elimination or freedom from it, but simply having changed its state, from solid to gas and making it even more dangerous not only for the environment but also for **human health.** All the energy of the second industrial revolution is based on the violation of the laws of thermodynamics. The combustion of a fuel to bring about propulsion or the turning of turbines is a thermodynamic folly with lethal consequences to human health. Changing the paradigm from the fossil cycle to the solar cycle, therefore entails activating a new, less harmful economy, consequently more in line with an illness prevention policy and closer to the objective of **zero disease.**

The Third Industrial Revolution is creating healthier and cleaner societies, an agriculture without pesticides or genetically modified organisms (GMO), a distributed industry instead of one centralized on **very reduced emissions.** On the contrary, continuing with the vertical logic will inevitably produce health **pollution** as an effect of soil, water and waste landfills contamination and the poisoning of air by incinerators.

However, with his new book, Rifkin causes us to reflect , he also covers the correlations between environment and health, he illuminates us on how the doctor/patient relation is changing in the dynamic of a new community of distributed health. Rifkin reaches this considerable result described also as the "**Commons of Health**".

Why not imagine, in fact, beyond the Commons of Information, the Commons of Energy, also the Commons of Health? "A Commons in which modern technologies of distributed and interactive information permit Dr Gille Frydman, founder of ACOR (**Association of Cancer Online resources**) to develop a model of participative medicine in which different subjects converge in a sole Commons. Patients, researchers, doctors, financers, producers of medical equipment, therapists, pharmaceutical companies and health professionals, would all be committed in collaborating to improve the care of the patient" (Rifkin, Society at Zero Marginal Cost, page 343).

This is not a remote or an unrealistic hypothesis. "Patientslikeme", a social network of over 200,000 e-patients already fights 1,800 diseases. An important achievement they have obtained has been exposing the scandal of lithium-based pharmaceuticals used for Amyotrophic Lateral Sclerosis. A study based on information received online showed how these drugs were totally uninfluential in the treatment against ALS. Such an example shows how the "open source" approach in **medical research** can produce important results, as opposed to competitive research, through which data remains trapped under a vertical, limited and secretive system.

In medicine, more than in any other sector, it becomes increasingly fundamental to dispose of "**big data**" with adequate algorithms, following the **crowdsourcing** model in order to identify sanitary models at low marginal costs and yet with very high efficiency. In the chapter "Everyone is a doctor" of his latest book, Jeremy Rifkin reminds us that, nowadays, the Internet counts with hundreds of health Open Source Commons. Rifkin consequently highlights that "everything suggests that their number will increase significantly in the coming years, when in various countries the electronic storage of health data will make health care support services more fluid and efficient... The big data, that will therefore be made possible to generate in the United States as in all other countries, will form a pool of information that, if properly exploited by open source Commons oriented health by patients, may, subject to appropriate safeguards on confidentiality, revolutionize the health sector" (Rifkin, Ibidem, page 348) .

Hence, the message launched from the collective of sensitive and intelligent doctors interpreting Rifkinian thought, among whom are Dr. Angela Meggiolaro, Dr Bruno Corda and Dr Angelo Barbato, **completes the vision** of a society of zero emissions, waste, kilometres and of a zero marginal cost economy.

The "Zero" vision expressed in the book-manifesto Zero Zone, written by professor Livio de Santoli and myself, thanks to the contribution of Angelo Barbato, has permitted us to trigger the spread of awareness around the **Zero Disease** concept. This occurs in a scenery in which the internet of things and the Third Industrial Revolution bring the centre of health care precisely onto the territory, calling for the necessity to increase prevention as a "Pillar" of the distributive model of health in medicine in the zone.

The new vision highlights that the traditional model based in the hospital has become ineffective for the treatment of **chronic diseases** which are increasingly diffused due to the lifestyles and occupations imposed since the Second Industrial Revolution, and which can be reduced by enhancing the prevention pillar. Telemedicine, home care, fight against chronic diseases, doctor's actions on the territory's schools and public administrations and especially the adoption of proactive methods by the citizen-patients, will increasingly revolutionize how we deal with health, moving the focus **from the institution to the area.**

This new health model of the third Industrial Revolution **will revolutionize the current paradigms of health care,** reaching extraordinary and very rapid results, mainly through prevention. The new care model is the heart of the book 'Zero Disease'. The realization of such a possible future depends entirely on us, starting from public administrations and health care enterprises. Notwithstanding citizens and their propulsive aggregating force which lead increasingly rapidly towards a biospheric, empathic, collaborative and sustainable lifestyle, where Community becomes Zero Zone.

Angelo Consoli
Director of the European Office of Jeremy Rifkin
President of CETRI-TIRES (Third Industrial Revolution European Society)
Co-Author with Livio de Santoli of the Manifesto-book "Zero Zone".

1. The wellness and health management in the ideological framework of Jeremy Rifkin

Bruno Corda Angelo Barbato

Jeremy Rifkin is one of the world's most recognized economists who in his recent work[1][2] has stressed the progressive rise of a new economic system, gradually alternating and replacing capitalism. The engine of this transformation is the digital revolution, allowing the **internet of things**. Telecommunications' Internet of things (or, more properly, the Internet of Things or IoT), is a neologism referring to the extension of Internet to the world of objects and concrete places[3]. The internet of things is made up of a network between the energy internet, the communication internet and the logistics internet[4]. Rifkin summarizes his economic thinking in three basic paradigms (energy, communications and logistics), stating that in the evolutionary change of these archetypes, man becomes the star of a new industrial revolution.

The first industrial revolution (about 1760-1870) was an economic transformation process or industrialization of society in which the agricultural and craft-trade systems became modernized and industrialized. Characterized by the generalized use of power-driven machines and of new, inanimate energy sources (such as fossil fuels - steam engines), the scheme was favored by a strong component of technological innovation. This was addi-

---

1 La società a costo marginale zero. L'Internet delle cose, l'ascesa del Commons Collaborativo e l'eclissi del capitalismo, Milano, Mondadori, 2014. ISBN 978-88-04-63980-0

2 La terza rivoluzione industriale. Come il "potere laterale" sta trasformando l'energia, l'economia e il mondo, Milano, Mondadori, 2011. ISBN 978-88-04-61420-3

3 https://it.wikipedia.org/wiki/Internet_delle_cose consulted 25 agosto 2015

4 https://it.wikipedia.org/wiki/Rivoluzione_industriale consulted 28 luglio 2015

tionally accompanied by the phenomena of growth, economic development and profound socio-cultural and even political changes. This first industrial revolution began in the textile (cotton), metallurgical (iron) and mining (hard coal) industries.

The insurgence of the **second industrial revolution** (about 1870-1970) is conventionally set to 1870 with the introduction of electricity, chemicals and oil.

The **third industrial revolution** (1970) refers to the effects of mass introduction into industry of electronics, telecommunications and informatics[5].

In recent years a new generation of scholars and specialists have began to realize that the management and centralized control of commerce is giving way to peer production and horizontal distribution. The scale of property exchange on the market is becoming less important than access to goods and services on the network. Additionally, conscience is rising around the **social capital as** true economic value rather than the market capital.

The main result will be a more equitable society based on sharing and cooperation between citizens and a sustainable economic model, particularly from an environmental point of view.

The new paradigm will lead to a progressive market decline as we know it today, parallel to the development of a **sharing economy** based on the cooperation of the consumer who meanwhile also becomes producer (prosumer). This is the first new economic system to make its appearance since the birth of capitalism and socialism at the beginning of the 1800. A free economy is emerging, a mix between capitalism and collaboration. In 2050 Jeremy Rifkin predicts that capitalism will still exist, but it won't be the sole economic system. Young people today collaborate with all sorts of things, produce and share their videos, their music, their news.

Online training courses are open and free, all this with

---

5 Stefano Battilossi, Le rivoluzioni industriali, Carocci, Roma, 2002, ISBN 88-430-2158-3

marginal costs equal to zero. In fact, when producing a video, the marginal cost to distribute it to a billion people is virtually zero.

We're starting to see a new economic system in which there aren't only producers and consumers, owners and workers but also **prosumers;** millions of people who access the Internet platforms of things and are able to produce, consume and share any virtual service: news, knowledge, music, video. We are by-passing the great twentieth-century organizations at almost zero marginal cost: free of charge, in abundance and outside the market. This is a revolution.

What will happen to **Multinationals**?

Many of the big and vertical ones of the twentieth-century have already been **destroyed,** as has happened, is occurring and will continue to take place in the music and video industry, in editorials and in television.

At the same time, thousands of other new **companies** have emerged in the economy **of sharing**. Not just Google, Facebook and Twitter, but thousands of profit and nonprofit companies that are building the sharing economy, thereby enabling young people to share what they create.

It 'a very destructive process to the market economy as we know it today, but it is only the beginning of a revolution towards the **democratization of economic life.**

Germany is leading this revolution, and even small countries like Denmark and Costa Rica are doing well. Germany is ahead in the internet of energy with 27% of the energy produced by sun and wind. It will be over 35% by 2020 and 100% by 2040. The costs of technologies for energy production are significantly reducing as has happened in the computer industry. A solar watt costed $ 150 in 1970, now it's charged 64 cents and it will drop to 35 within 18 months. Once Germany has paid off the investment expenses, the marginal cost of energy produced will be close to zero. The sun and the wind do not send any bill to be paid to the Germans. It's free. Germany is heading towards an energy system at zero marginal cost that will make the economy more productive and efficient in the world, hugely benefitting its businesses and families.

China, too, has begun to change its energy policy with investments starting at 82 billion dollars in 2015 to digitize the electric grid smart. Millions of Chinese will be able to produce solar and wind energy in their home and share it in the national electricity grid.

In electrical engineering and telecommunications, a **smart grid (intelligent network)** is the combination of an information network and an electrical distribution network in a manner allowing to manage the power grid "smartly".

Precisely the **"intelligent" characteristic** must be highlighted under various aspects or features as the efficient distribution of electrical energy for its more rational use, minimizing any overloads and variations in voltage around its nominal value[6].

Digital smart grid is a concept which, carried from the power supply, will be increasingly developed in the computer network connections. This has implications not only for Wi-Fi, broadband and big data. It is needed to move towards the trend of digitizing the three major paradigms of the economy: energy, communications and logistics (including transport systems).

There are no longer virtual or natural boundaries facing the great global problems such as population growth, food resources, over-exploitation of land resources, pollution of the planet and consequently uncontrolled problems at the limit of survival , of space and of the **biosphere's** balance. These represent problems towards which consciousness is growing, issues we can no longer postpone, or worse, ignore.

A new global and social consciousness is inevitably making its way, demanding a complete change of paradigms. Vertical and power relations will gradually give way to relations of **cooperation and sharing** of forces.

---

6 https://it.wikipedia.org/wiki/Smart_grid consulted 13 ottobre 2015

Empathy and assertiveness, keywords of sharing and collaboration, will integrate the necessarily narcissistic, closed and conservative communities of all sizes and places.

As masterfully described by Jeremy Rifkin, history shows that a shift in **energy, communication and logistics** represents the dawn of a substantial economic revolution in all societies of the world. Consequently, as always happens during great changes, it is crucial for the future of society to seize the opportunities of such shifts, renewing and adapting their inner world to a new global vision. At present, the history of man and of civilization has reached a global dimension.

The paradigmatic events of the third industrial revolution described by Jeremy Rifkin have produced the greatest **evolutionary acceleration** in human history. As always, it is up to man to know how to seize new opportunities. The faster man makes this happen, the deeper and more aware the willingness to change themselves will be.

The first big change is radical, the gradual transition from a self-centered individual awareness to an **open and multifocal collective**. In summary, the ability to combine oneself with others and with the surrounding world is needed. This three-dimensional view, which effectively defines the so-called biosphere consciousness is the new interior condition absolutely necessary to be able to rapidly take advantage of the great benefits that this revolutionary global process can generate.

Not knowing how to seize this great opportunity, or worse, not wanting to participate in the change can result in **unfavorable social events**, which are already perceivable, if not visible.

History is continually proposing this.

Individuals and companies are therefore becoming increasingly collaborative, more involved, more empathetic, more attentive to the world in which they live in. The **change** will impact our lives more rapidly the more we are active participants.

This will happen in the production of goods, but above all

in the collective sphere of relations, so-called **services**. First and foremost, is **health,** where the value of empathy is one of the anchors of the modern conception of the doctor-patient relationship.

The **doctor-patient relationship** has always been the cornerstone and the centerpiece of the "cure" process in all its stages, from prevention to diagnosis to therapy.

In some national contexts, such liaison has gradually shifted towards the establishment of mathematical sterile space protocols of production chain in the Health "**Companies**", sometimes operated by speculative organizations. These companies are both public and private. Speculative, in this context, because the "enterprises", rather than focusing on the "production of health", end up feeding themselves and their survival.

Why are the delivery systems for health care services continually reviewed? What is constantly changing? Why do public health systems tend towards privatization and not vice- versa? Why is an important profession such as health care more than any other at the centre of debates and controversies? Why is one of the most important services that every state should give priority to so different from country to country?

The evolution of society has gradually shifted its focus to the level of the hierarchy of needs, as has inevitably been the case also for one of the basic services organized for citizens in modern societies, "**health protection**".

Today, the **close individual-environment connection** is undeniable, seeing the correlations between environmental degradation and health risks. This awareness has been gradually triggering growing consciousness and the culture of prevention.

The environmental crisis, the crisis of health and the crisis of values are closely linked and interdependent. The system responds to the request for health with an increasing number of expensive and technologically sophisticated performances; trying to modify the natural history of "disease", which in itself already implies "lost health". Neglecting, instead, primary **prevention** which is to be made both on the polluted and unhealthy environment around us, as well as on individuals, accompanied by an appropriate policy of information and health education in search of a more simple and sustainable lifestyle.

Ethical and social values are sometimes contrasted by **economic value**, hence the need to make the health system sustainable while ensuring conditions of equality and universality.

All countries in the world are committed to finding answers for the enhancement of its citizens' health.

Various countries, principally the developed ones, have established health care management models essentially of two types: a predominantly public model named **Beveridge** after the Englishman who at the end of World War II brought public insurance coverage to the United Kingdom, the "National Health Service"; and the **Bismarck** model, which takes its name from the Prussian/German statesman who introduced the private health insurance system.

Different countries have tried, even with customizations, to adjust such organizational models to the ever-changing demand for health, in the variable environmental and economic contexts, in order to maximize their population's health.

In the 90's, the **World Health Organization** altered the attention level of health protection systems, shifting attention from the treatment of diseases, to seeking the psychological **well-being** of individuals and the environmental determinants of health.

To organize health care, man began his fight against diseases that in the nineteenth century was focused on therapies against infectious diseases. Around 1850, the construction of the first **pavilion hospitals** began, which soon showed the potential of hosting and connecting specialized activities that were beginning to emerge. These were mostly surgical, as a result of the revolutionary scientific discoveries and practices of the birth era of the foundations for anesthesia, microbiology, antisepsis and asepsis, but also diagnostic laboratory support, followed by diagnostic radiology (X-ray, 1901 Nobel prize), to which electrocardiographic diagnostics[7] would be added soon after (Einthoven, 1908).

In order to organize health care in addition to acute patient management and thus urgency/ emergency, you need an increasing ability to manage **chronic illness** through a holistic vision that includes active handling of the disease, more often chronic diseases to be centered on **prevention.**

In recent years the traditional and hierarchical health care model that is identified with hospital care has began to falter, not only due to the high cost of energy, technology and management but also because of the profound epidemiological changes in diseases. Traditionally, the cure of acute illnesses has reportedly developed a **standby medicine** in the top-down hospital context, a facility increasingly dedicated to users, emergency and to the treatment of high intensity and in need of advanced technologies. The hospital has become ineffective for the treatment of rising widespread chronic diseases in need of multidimensional interventions, also linked with social health.

The increase in **life expectancy** with the progressive ageing of the population has led to the augmentation of chronic degenerative and debilitating diseases, for which the traditional hospital standby model is inadequate.

The attempt to create within the **hospital outpatient sectors** for specialized external uses has proved **unsuccessful** for a number of reasons: the structural and hospital management costs are too high for such activities, and the type of performance is completely different since the acute patient must be treated in the hospital and the chronically ill should be treated in the zone, through the enhancement of organizational models characterized by prevention.

Merging the management of activities for acute disease with the management of the activities for chronic illness inside

---

7 E. Guzzanti: L'ospedale del futuro: origini, evoluzione, prospettive. Recenti progressi in medicina Vol. 97, N. 11, Novembre 2006 Pagg. 594-603

the hospital deviates high-tech and urgency resources from interventions for the acutely ill. The center of gravity of care for chronic conditions needs to be moved into the territory, with the need for increased effectiveness also through avoidance interventions. **Prevention** becomes **the pillar of the distributive model** of territorial health care: not only due to its undisputed importance in the promotion and maintenance of health, but also for the better utilization of resources, resulting in cost reduction. The new strategies for the integration of health policies must necessarily take into account **environmental sustainability**.

After a period of constant evolution and adaptation of the specific structure for increasingly accurate, effective, technically advanced and prognostically favorable treatments, - **the hospital** - the focus, has opened itself towards the territorial zone for several reasons.

The **hospital** is a highly sophisticated structure with high technological trends, high management costs only justifiable for performance-intensive care given to a patient in acute emergency and made possible only in a protected environment.

The **territory** consequently gains importance not only to provide care and treatment to low-intensity patients and to guarantee care continuity and the patient's recovery. But above all, to prevent and anticipate the disease (early detection!). In addition, the territory also represents an important input filter and selector for hospitalization.

The **hospital**, by vocation, treats (or should treat!) **100% of the acutely ill**, while health outside the hospital treats (or should treat!) mainly the healthy to ensure a minimal occurrence of sickness.

The **primary care target** is therefore made up of 40% of healthy individuals, 40% of healthy individuals with risk factors and the remaining 20% of ill individuals (of which 10% have disabilities).

The hospital's **mission** is maximum repair and cure of the individual's biological damage, while the mission of the zone is to avoid health damage through multiple strategies on population health, even informing and educating people of the best way to live .

In a distributed model of medicine of the territory, health professionals and family physicians are the central figures in order to achieve a proactive medicine. **Proactive medicine** is centered on the promotion of good health and the prevention of bad health. The health of a community is determined by socioeconomic and environmental factors, lifestyle and access to services. It is evident that only the model of distributed medicine in the territory with a central role in prevention can ensure the implementation of a wide range of initiatives, projects and policies necessary for effective health promotion.

Hence, the necessity emerges for an integrated strategy between governmental bodies and non-governmental bodies, in the possible fields for regional action. From the action of doctors on the territory and in schools, to interventions by the public authorities through training activities based on epidemiological evidence. The concept of integration is essential and must be developed in a distributed **model of Zero Zone**, cornerstones of which is home medicine and telemedicine: i.e. trying to bring care closer to the patient-citizen.

Modern medicine (with the exception of acute illnesses) should become "**initiative-based**", since it must not be the citizen-patient to contact the hospital system but the Zero Zone to take the burden of health in a proactive manner by trying to prevent the development of chronic disease. Proactive medicine has the primary objective of avoiding the disease (primary interception with its information tools, health education, empowerment, control and information on the risk factors). Secondly, its tasks are early recognition of onset pathological conditions (secondary prevention) through targeted interventions and rapid, highly qualified, epidemiological study and monitoring of collective health, determinants of well-being and illness.

To **develop the model of Zero Zone**, synonymous of active and preventive approach, multidisciplinary, integrated, non-hierarchical, structured network; high computerization (internet of things) is required. Among the tools in exponential development we find apps, increasingly becoming key elements in the communication between doctor and patient (bidirectional energy binomial), essential for effective therapeutic action thanks to i thets significant synergistic effect.

The sustainability of the health system in a distributed model that can not be separated from an integration with the **social** in the Zero Zone logic (sharing economy).

ZERO Zone is simultaneously a basic and complex operation. The idea is simple: to program a society that tends towards zero entropy. The work to get there is complex since it involves new mental paradigms, new educational models, new business strategies, new administrative measures. Examples are the overcoming of departments of energy, economic development, environment, agriculture, in favor of departments to commons goods or land resources. Smart grids are the digital infrastructures of the Internet of things that allow the connection between energy, communications and logistics. In electrical engineering and telecommunications, a smart grid represents the combining of an information network and an electrical distribution network in such a way as to allow the management of the electrical network in an"intelligent" manner under various aspects or features. In other words, the efficient distribution of electrical energy and a more rational use of energy; thereby minimizing any overloads and variations of the voltage around its nominal value[8].

According to the ideological picture of Jeremy Rifkin, a **distributed model** (Commons) should be applied to the way in which food and energy are produced and the creation of polluting waste at the end of the fuel cycle is avoided. According to the authors, this also concerns the way in which health care is organized in the territory, through the distributed pillar of prevention

---

8 https://it.wikipedia.org/wiki/Smart_grid consulted 24 agosto 2015

(**Zero Disease**) which can only be formed in the Commons. The smart grid digital health is thus being born.

In "The zero marginal cost society" Jeremy Rifkin argues that a new economic system is emerging on the world stage, the rise of the Internet of things is giving life to the "**Collaborative Commons**", the first new economic paradigm to take hold by the advent of capitalism and socialism in the nineteenth century. Collaborative Commons is transforming the way we co-ordinate economic life opening up the possibility to a drastic reduction in income inequality by democratizing the global economy and creating a more environmentally sustainable society.

In a distributed scenario of the Third Industrial Revolution, it is unimaginable to think of a health care model based on concentration as during the second industrial revolution, which must therefore be overcome once and for all by introducing **prevention** practices across the geographical zone.

It can not be said that a public health system of a state or region (**model "Beveridge"**) is always better than a private health care system of a state or region (**model "Bismarck"**).

On the contrary, states or regions, in order to have an efficient and effective health service must put in place a model where public and private sectors are in **competition** with each other.

The ideological framework of Jeremy Rifkin sees three basic paradigms (energy, communications and logistics) complementing each other in a hierarchical and top-down economy, evolving **distributively** through cost-sharing economic systems. health care is a service, and as such tends to evolve towards the sharing economy and collaborative community (commons).

In the social model indicated by Jeremy Rifkin, can health services also be **alternatives** to the two historical organizational models of Bismarck and Beveridge?

Even for health services, it emerges that, to appropriately meet the growing and new health requirements, it is necessary to improve the economic system with the best cost/ benefit ratio and the lowest possible entropy. The new route also in health care is the development of the economy of sharing and the development of collaborative communities (commons) where the comparison between institutions, citizens and health specialists will be revolutionized by a new patient-citizen as an increasingly active element and aware of his rights. The intelligent digital networks for health will spread increasingly (**Health Smart grid Digital**).

The fundamental paradigms of intelligent digital networks for health, which set the new model, correspond to a **complementarity between the paradigms** of a Zero Zone oriented towards a society at a zero marginal cost, with Zero Disease turned towards an exponential contrast of the disease with an ideal trend of making it null.

ZERO ZONE	ZERO DISEASE
ENERGY	HEALTHY BEINGS
COMMUNICATION	DOCTOR/PATIENT RELATIONSHIP (role of internet in prevention and prediction)
LOGISTICS	HEALTHCARE (management)

Jeremy Rifkin's prediction is applicable not only to the production of all goods and to all **services** but even more importantly to service excellence in the protection of health.

The paradigm of energy Zero Zone finds reciprocity with the **maintenance of health (to be healthy)**, of zero disease .

The paradigm of Zero Zone communication finds reciprocity in the **evolution of the doctor/ patient relationship** through the development of the internet and the strengthening of preventive medicine and predictive zero disease.

The archetype of Zero Zone logistics bares reciprocity in the organizational model of health management (**healthcare**).

Even in **healthcare** a third way will come to develop through the use of specific energy elements (consciousness biospheric), communication (empathy, empowerment and assertiveness) and health care logistics; the health Commons or the sharing economy and collaborative communities (commons).

2. Historical evolution of healthcare assistance

2.1 From Hippocrates to the discovery of antibiotics

Hippocrates was born in Greece in **460 B.C.** and died also in Greece in **377 B.C.** He is considered the father of medicine. Treating disease and the sick has been a necessity formed with the very origin of man; as a spontaneous need of the patient to live in the community while not being alone against an illness. "*Medicus*" is not only the one who mediates between the patient and the disease, but also who stands between evil and death, often taking over the centuries a mystic or priestly role. The first medical schools were developed in the area of present-day Greece and Ancient Greece, including in Sicily and Calabria. In Crotone, Calabria, the school of **Pythagoras (570 BC - 495 BC)**[9] was famous. At the center of the Hippocratic conception there was not the disease but rather a man with an extreme attention towards nutrition and the environment. This was the precursor of the knowledge of the first determinants of disease related to nutrition and healthy air. The writings of Hippocrates (or assumed so) were analyzed in the universities until the 1700. Such manuscripts were oriented towards prudence and caution before intervening with the moderate use of therapy also since in those days there were few remedies available, pharmacology was not yet known and herbal medicine was in its infancy, growing about a century later with **Theophrastus (371 B.C. - 287 B.C.)**, a pupil of **Aristotle (384 B.C. - 322 B.C.)** to whom we owe an enormous boost of natural sciences.

Hippocrates gave medicine a holistic imprint centred on man and the environment, becoming in fact the precursor of the most advanced modern environmentalist theories, including the

---

9 http://pacs.unica.it/biblio/storia1.htm consultato il 21 giugno 2015

economic and ecological ones of our economist of reference, Jeremy Rifkin: our guide in describing the new paradigm of medicine that with this paper we disseminate: Zero Disease.

Hippocrates introduced the first concepts of medical ethics and it is to his school that the **doctor's oath** is attributed:

- *"I swear by Apollo the healer, by Asclepius, by Hygieia, by Panacea, and by all the Gods and Goddesses, making them my witnesses, that I will carry out, according to my ability and judgment, this oath: I swear to to honour like I honour my parents he who taught me the art of medicine (concept of pupil-teacher); to share with him my sustainment and satisfy his needs, if he may need it;*

- *to consider his sons as my own brothers, and to teach them this art, if they want to learn it, without fee or indenture;*

- *to impart precept, oral instruction, and all other instruction to my own sons, the sons of my teacher, and to indentured pupils who have taken the physician's oath, but to nobody else (concept of caste);*

- *I will apply the diet regime for the advantage of the ill, according to my ability and judgement, I will spread them against anything harmful and unjust;*

- *I will not administer a poison to anybody when asked to do so, nor will I suggest such a course. Similarly I will not give to a woman a pessary to cause abortion;*

- *I will keep pure and holy both my life and my profession. I will not operate on who sufferers from stone, and will leave such practice to professionals;*

- *"Into whatever house I enter, it will be to help the sick, and I will abstain from all intentional corruption, especially from seducing women, men, free and slaves. And whatsoever I shall see or hear in the exercise of my profession as well as outside my profession that I can hear or see regarding the life of others that should not be divulged, I shall tacite, holding such things as secrets (concept of professional secret);*

- *I carry out this oath all the way and honour it, may I be able to enjoy the fruits of my life and of this art, forever honoured by all men; but if I transgress it and forswear myself, may the opposite befall me".*

Hygiene, from greek "*salutare*", is the branch of medicine that deals with health in a holistic way from its earliest conception that studies the wholesomeness of air, soil and water to its most **modern conception** that studies how to organize in public and private health care the health services as efficiently and effectively as possible. Hygiene has always dealt with how to prevent disease.

Democritus (460 B.C. - 370 B.C.) developed the theory of pores that came to condition the scarcity of hygiene that was found in the Middle Ages. For the school of Democritus, depending on whether the pores were open or closed, there would have been a condition respectively of relaxation or tension. According to this theory, it was necessary to try to maintain the pores naturally open with resulting attention on how to wash and on the water temperature. This concept was misinterpreted in the Middle Ages condemning water as a cause for the closure of the pores.

Fortunately, the erroneous theories of Democritus were uptaken only many centuries later (Middle Ages) while during the Greek and Roman era there was a remarkable development of hygiene. The **water** was the **key element of Roman society** that allowed the realization of impressive aqueducts passing through the streets of the empire and considerable construction of spas and saunas with an advanced water and sewage system.

The contrast to *infectious diseases* was conducted over the centuries especially thanks to the **different hygiene techniques** that, as we will see, will lead to the development of *preventive medicine* to the very recent *predictive medicine* and *personalized medicine*.

To fight diseases, medical facilities with a high concentration doctors and technology called **hospitals**, have developed over the past centuries. The modern hospital's origins can be traced back to the early twentieth century and initially it was the wealthy landowners who left a will in favor of places that dealt with poor and dying patients. These were charitable structures, almost always managed and organized by religious people.

Despite the catastrophic plague pandemics and raged **leprosy** and **tuberculosis** of the fourteenth and seventeenth centuries there was no awareness that the disease could be contagious to another living organism. The modes of transmission of infectious diseases were unknown and the most accepted theory was that odors carried the contagion, but no one knew how. In the Middle Ages there was no concept of hygiene and the sick were put on the beds with dirty sheets that was recycled without washing.

The **hospital** of the first industrial revolution can be traced back to the **eighteenth century**, a large and promiscuous operation between social and health care, where febrile patients were hospitalized with women in childbirth, psychiatric cases, surgical patients at risk of nosocomial gangrene but also the poor in need of shelter and food.

With the rise of environmental health knowledge to counter **infectious diseases** the pavilion hospital model began its development, built with low buildings separated from each other to avoid to a maximum contagion from one patient to another. Around 1850 began the construction of the first hospitals in pavilions that can still be seen today in the center of ancient metropolitan cities such as the Umberto I General Hospital and the San Camillo Hospital in Rome.

Gerolamo Fracastoro (1478 - 1553)[10] doctor, mathematician and poet, taught logic in the University of Padua. He wrote the latin poem *Syphilis sive de morbo gallico* (1530), which tells of a young and handsome shepherd who, having offended Apollo, is punished with a terrible ulcerative colitis. Syphilis, a venereal disease at the time newly spreading, took its name from this poem. Fracastoro was among the first to believe that epidemic diseases were transmitted by a sort of seminal entity that carries the contagion (*De contagione et contagiosis morbis*, 1546).

Carlo Francesco Cogrossi (1682-1769) was the first who noticed that bovine plague had living organisms that transmitted the plague, but his argument fell on deaf ears.

Edward Jenner (1749-1823) was a british naturalist and doctor, know for introducing the vaccine against smallpox and considered the father of immunization.

The use of certain molds and plants for the cure of infections was already recognized in ancient cultures- greek, egyptian, chinese - their effectiveness was due to **antibiotic substances** produced by the vegetale species or by the mold. However, there was no possibility to distinguish the effectively active component nor isolate it. Vincenzo Tiberio, Molisane doctor in the University of Naples, already in 1895 described the antibacterial power of

---

10 http://www.chieracostui.com/costui/docs/search/scheda.asp?ID=2661 consultato 10 agosto 2015

some molds[11].

Modern research began with **Alexander Flemming's** casual on penicillin in 1928. More than ten years later, **Ernst Chain** and **Howard Walter Florey** managed to obtain antibiotics in pure form. The three obtained for their merits the Nobel Prize for medicine in 1945.

---

11 Gli antibiotici? Una scoperta italiana, almanacco.rm.cnr.it. consultato 10 agosto 2015

2.2. The healthcare systems: public (welfare state and Beveridge) and private (Bismark)

Bruno Corda, Angelo Barbato, Angela Meggiolaro

The welfare state is based on the principle of equality and characterizes the modern states of law. The rights and the welfare state guaranteed services are basically **health care**, public education and social security. The ordinances of the nations with a greater development of the welfare state also provide greater investment and programs for the defense of the natural environment and unemployment benefits (citizen income).

The health care models are essentially two: a mutualistic system (**Bismarck**) based on private appeal and a National Health Service (**Beveridge**) with public and universal vocation.

In relation to the **welfare state** of the post-war Europe until the 80s, four main areas can be classified: Scandinavia, Anglo-Saxon, Continental Europe and Southern Europe. Although for large schematization it can be said that historically the north of Europe as a matrix refers to the universal model (Beveridge) while continental Europe and southern historically is characterized as originally mutualistic (Bismarck).

Scientific and popular literature offer a wide variety of treaties on the **History of Public Health**, providing a definitely eclectic and comprehensive view on the various aspects and focus areas. In 1989, Mullan wrote about the history of public health in the US; Duffy in 1992 focused on the work of Health Care Workers; Fee in 2002 has followed a wide variety of articles on the historical aspects of public health while Warner and Tighe in 2006 have emphasized the link between Public Health and Clinical Medicine[12].

In ancient civilizations, public health was geared exclusively towards the protection of **public hygiene**. During the Roman Empire, the care of the poor sick was entrusted to archiatrists paid by the city. The creation of the first hospital-like struc-

---

12 Fallon, L. F., & Zgodzinski, E. J. (2005). Essentials of public health management. Jones & Bartlett Learning

tures dates back to the Middle Ages: they were centers who had a more charitable rather than health purpose, in fact the first institutions of its kind developed in the vicinity of bishoprics, monasteries and along pilgrimage routes[13].

During the **Renaissance** the first attempt of a systematic classification of diseases was undertaken; while during the Enlightenment took place the first investigation of diseases and of the overall health of the population. The French Revolution and the **first industrial revolution** (about 1760-1870) with the consequent urbanization, contributed to giving a strong incentive to the concept of public health.

The **Health Movement** has been a product of the **second industrial revolution**, a new approach to public health developed in England between 1830 and 1840. With the growing industrialization and urbanization, increasing awareness about the importance of personal hygiene and the human waste treatment has led as a strategic choice in the fight against infectious diseases to sanitation and removal of filth from the cities. However, as understood by Edwin Chadwick, urban cleaning in the literal sense, has become, over time, a deviant figurative meaning, and was seen as the removal of a potential health threat represented by "dangerous classes." Other European cities such as Paris and Naples followed suit, undertaking reconstruction projects on a large scale. However, these technological reforms marked an undeniable step forward for public health, often leading to the exclusion of economic and educational reforms[14].

The concept of Public Health, therefore, has over time expanded its scope of application and interest, taking shape first as **action towards the Community** for the prevention of diseases and threats to health, for the wellbeing of individuals and the

---

13 http://www.treccani.it/enciclopedia/sanita-pubblica_(Dizionario-di-Storia)/ultimo accesso: 1 ottobre 2015

14 http://oyc.yale.edu/history/hist-234/lecture-11_HIST 234 consultato 1 novembre 2015 EPIDEMICS IN WESTERN SOCIETY SINCE 1600Lecture 11 - The Sanitary Movement and the "Filth Theory of Disease" Overview

population; successively reaching to include both the promotion and the protection of health[15].

In the eighteenth century, in **Europe**, the organization of Public Health was the exclusive competence of judicial and police organs with tasks limited to the management of epidemics and outbreaks.

In **England**, the British factory act is approved for the regulation of the workloads in factories (1833) and in 1948 the NHS (National Health Service) is founded. Doctors of Public Health were appointed: the Medical Officer of Health.

Surprisingly, it is up to **America** to lead the first attempt to establish a Health System of Universalistic nature, extended to the majority of the population. In 1910 C. Chapin wrote what later became the reference text of the 'Public Health', not only American.

Appearing between the lines of the ideal of a Public Health, is not only 'science and art of preventing disease' but also the promotion of a quality of life, preservation and extension of the state of health and physical efficiency. In that sense, the **participatory role of the entire community** becomes fundamental. In this model of **'distributed'** Public Health, the community becomes, albeit with still a passive role, starring in ensuring the maintenance of adequate living standards, appropriate for the extension of health conditions. Among the main action lines of the document was education of the patient on common preventive measures, the elementary rules of hygiene, and the promotion of environmental health.

Public Health therefore becomes 'Health System', beginning to take a tangible organizational configuration and initially structured in centers of power and control and in systems of provision of health actions. Just as we will see later in the historical

---

15 Origini e sviluppo della sanità pubblica Sanità pubblica http://www.sociologia.uniroma1.it/users/tarsitani/storia%20sanit%C3%A0%20pubb%20SSN.pdf consultato 1 novembre 2015

evolution of these public models in different countries, the inability to keep separate and distinct the commissioners' roles (the centres of power and control) and the role of the regulator has heavily contributed to the crisis of the system.

Currently, the concept of **New Public Health** [16]is emerging, according to which health is an investment in the life of the community. The New Public Health focuses on the behavior of individuals in their environment and the conditions that influence such behavior.

The **application fields** of public health include not only the scientific, but also the social, cultural and political spheres.

In addition to the classic notion of disease prevention, the work of Public Health is dedicated to **promoting** physical and mental **health** of individuals. Those objectives are reflected in trying to influence the habits and living conditions, but also in promoting self-esteem, human dignity and respect.

Public Health is the set of actions undertaken by the company to improve the **health** of a population.

A commonly accepted classification of health systems is based on the terms of financing and is distinguished between **insurance-based systems** (Social Health Insurance) and **tax-based systems** (general taxation).

The more established **Health Systems** in Europe are: the Beveridge model, the Bismarck model, the Mixed model and the Semasko model.

While the last two have hybrid features, among the **first two** substantial differences can be identified.

The mixed model instead provides for the simultaneous presence of taxation mechanisms and forms of social insurance, providing coverage of the entire population.

The **Semasko model**, finally, is typical of those countries which currently or in the past decade have seen a political and

---

16
http://www.eupha.org/documents/publications/eupha_10_statements_(italian).pdf consultato 25 agosto 2015

social environment in transition (Central Europe and the former Soviet Union). This system is similar to the Bismarck model for the connotations related to social insurance mechanisms, even though it is funded by directly withholding tax on salary.

In the **Beveridge model**, health systems are primarily financed through tax revenues and should provide all of the services. The taxation may be direct or indirect, national or local.

The British National Health Service, or **NHS**, was founded in 1948 in order to provide free healthcare to the entire population of Britain. It is the first National Health System of the Beveridge style: universal, free, financed by general taxation[17].

A first attempt of de-verticalization of the healthcare system took place in Britain in 1990 with the 'NHS and Community Care Act', better known as the **Thatcher Reform.**

History, ever since the first reforms and the Darwinian evolution of the healthcare system would not seem to have favored vertically integrated organizational models, centralized or monocratic in the regulation of supply and demand, but have rather veered towards more **'distributed** forms' for the provision and management of health. In the specific case of the Thatcher Reform, this was targeted towards precise incentivizing objectives to enhance the efficiency of Services. Therefore the hierarchical and monolithic model was shattered in favor of a separationist approach between buyer and distributor, introducing competition mechanism between producers; nevertheless maintaining the underlying principles of solidarity financing and access to the proper services of a public system.

In the late '80s, the proposal of the economist Enthoven [1988] to reform European healthcare systems in the light of the US **HMO** integrated organizations meets the favor of **conservative governments**, such as Reagan and, precisely, Thatcher. With the reform of 1990, England adopts a quasi-market variant called the internal markets model, in which the competition between

---

17 http://www.sochealth.co.uk/national-health-service/reform-of-the-national-health-service/ consultato 27 agosto 2015

public or private producers is enabled by special public agencies that act as patient representatives (sponsors) and, given a default loan, buy from producers through health services contracts for the assisted population. The idea of the quasi-market goes from England to the rest of Europe, with diverse applications in different European healthcare systems, oscillating between the two opposite poles of the total programming and pure market, thereby adopting intermediate hybrid forms of health care organization with various combinations of hierarchical mechanisms of control and competition[18].

In the **Bismarck** model, born in Germany in <u>1883</u> and introduced by Chancellor <u>Otto von Bismarck</u> to help reduce the mortality and injury in the workplace and to establish an early form of social security, the systems are financed by social insurances. The private style Bismarck model is characterized, on one hand by contributions generally assessed based on salaries, and on the other hand the organizations, which are called Funds diseases, act as administrative structures of the system and payers for care. The number of funds and their size vary widely with respect to the number of members and their employment status. In most cases up to the government to determine the contribution rates. In some countries you can choose the fund to support, (as is the case for example in Germany, Holland, and Switzerland), in others not. As regards to the **German** health system we must go back in time, until January 18, 1871 at the time of birth of the German Empire or Deutsches Kaiserreich, the Second Reich, following the victory of Germany in both the Austro-Prussian and the Franco-Prussian wars. After which, comes a period characterized by a strong fear by the part of the monarchies of the various states that the French Revolution could also happen in Germany. German nationalism rapidly moves from its liberal and democratic character in 1848 to Otto von Bismarck's authoritar-

---

18 Saltman N, Richard B.; VON OTTER, Casten. Re-vitalizing public health care systems: a proposal for public competition in Sweden. Health Policy, 1987, 7.1: 21-40.&

ian Realpolitik, which uses the "carrot and stick approach". The socialist movement was banned, but an especially advanced welfare state is created; based on compulsory social insurance, financed by contributions from companies and workers. In 1883, insurance for illness is established, in 1884 for accidents on the workplace, in 1889 disability and old age pensions are institutionalized.

This created what was at the time the most advanced welfare system in the world. A model (Bismarck model) that became an example, since the early twentieth century, adopted in most of the industrialized countries and which still exists in Germany and other countries. An **expensive** model, since - after the US - in the Organisation for Economic Co-operation and Development (OECD) ranking regarding the percentage of GDP spent on health care (year 2012), appear all countries belonging to the Bismarck model, with Germany in 5th place with 11.3%.

The same applies to the **health expenditure per capita**, which is $ 4,811 in Germany in 2012 (of which $ 3,651 - 75.9% - public health expenditure). This represents a much lower cost than the one corresponding to the US ($ 8,745), but much higher than the OECD average ($ 3,484), or that of Britain ($ 3,289) and Italy ($ 3,209).

Following the **financial crisis of 2008**, Germany, parallelly to the average of the OECD countries, has seen a sharp slowdown in annual growth in health spending that from + 4% in 2008 rose to a little less than +1%, while other Southern European countries have suffered a net reduction of resources available in real terms: -2% Spain, Italy -3%, Portugal 6%, Greece -10%.

In terms of burdens on citizens, Germany spends a lot on health care, but still produces a huge amount of services, with a low level of direct spending by patients. This shows that we are faced with a technically efficient system.

The German population consists of 81.8 million citizens. The 85% of them are enrolled in one of the **132 social** "compulsory" **insurances** (Krankenkassen). These are "non-profit" insurances, "friendly societies", not definable as public, nor private. Until 1996 the inscription was attached to the profession; since then a liberalization has taken place, thereby allowing the possibility of choice between different insurance companies competing with each other for charges and coverings offered to its members.

The **registration requirement** applies to all employees (and their families) with a gross monthly income equal to or less than € 4462.60. It is the state itself that pays, through specific funding of the Länder, for assistance of the disabled, the unemployed, minors or for categories that otherwise can not subscribe to insurance.

The contribution paid to the Krankenkassen varies depending on the employee's income and corresponds to **15.5% of the monthly salary (53%** of which is paid by the **employee** and **47%** by the **employer**). Thus a financial equalization is applied to compensate for the different capacity of contribution of members: Each person pays proportionally to their income. The contribution of employees and businesses has grown over the past 15 years, going from 13.6% in 1998 to currently 15.5% of the monthly income.

On top of the monthly contribution, **supplements** (Zuzahlungen) are added: you have to pay € 10 every three months to take advantage of medical consultations with all doctors recognized by the health insurance funds, and thereafter each time that you are using one visit to the doctor or dentist (including those covered by the policy) you have to pay a fee of 10 € (this "Praxisgebühr" has led to an observed reduction of 10% of the accesses). Even for the medicines you pay 10% of the price, and 10 € per day for hospitalization. Recently, an annual limit for additional expenses has been set (generally 2% of annual income, 1% for recipients of a continuing care because of a serious chronic disease), those who pass such percentage are reimbursed their insurance. Minors do not pay any additional charge.

In Germany there is an **obligation** to be insured; those with a monthly income of more than € 4462.60 may choose to subscribe to private insurances (Private Krankenversicherung-PKV), rather than social ones.

Private insurances, unlike the mutualistic funds in which the contribution depends on income, calculate the premium depending on the **personal risk** (in fact, it is provided thorough medical examination before enrolling). Private insurances often offer superior services of social insurance, pay better doctors, and also offer reimbursements for hospitalization in non-contracted private clinics. For young people with a high salary and no health problem, the contribution towards the private enterprises often costs much less; with age the insurance policy increases in price. However, even in case of serious diseases it may not exceed certain standard levels (for this reason it is custom for young people to appeal to insurances to create a capital backup with their savings). Nine million Germans, equal to 11% of the population are privately insured. The use of private insurance can also be a complementary purpose for those who are enrolled in the Krankenkassen (about 23 million). The main reason is to expand the financial protection in case of illness or hospitalization. The remaining 4% of the population is represented by people who get insurance coverage through special channels, such as the military or those with refugee status.

The **funding of the German health system** is mainly based on the takings of the compulsory social insurance (57%) and on private insurances (9%). The central government is not involved in the health system neither as a financier nor as manager, or as the owner of sanitary manufacturing companies (except detailed cases, such as military hospitals). However, it governs the whole system, defining the rules by which the actors can move. Mutual aid societies and associations of physicians operate within administrative rules, only modifiable by the central government, just as they are regulated by laws and relations between the different actors of the system. Although the general health policies for the country are decided by the Central State, the management and the funding of the system takes place at regional level, where there are three institutions: the Land (through its Ministry of Health), mutual aid societies, associations of panel doctors and hospitals. It is the individual Länder who plan and finance investments and infrastructure (hospitals, departments, equipment, access to the conventions and specialized training), credit the volume of production, finance the hospital-area system integration and perform the review of legality. These can, for instance, control the activity of doctors and guide their prescription behavior towards less expensive drugs, as well as carry out surveillance on the quality of hospital care.

The sickness insurance funds programming negotiate and acquire the services for their patients. The German system's financing mechanism is therefore **dualistic**: the **Land** defines and funds investment, while the **mutual aid society** negotiates and finances the current healthcare costs by dealing with both hospitals and affiliated physicians.

For hospital functions, the regional association for mutual aid signs a **contract with each hospital**, while for **outpatient functions** it negotiate a global agreement with the **regional association of doctors**.

Mutual aid is called to protect the interests of its members, trying to influence the volume and the producer's case mix, as well as to respect the insurance spending thresholds, implicitly set out by the Government through the maximum rate of contributions payable by the subscribers.

With an excess of **hospital beds** (8.3 per 1,000 inhabitants compared to the OECD average of 4.8 and 2.6 in Sweden and 3.4 in Italy), the rate of hospitalization (25 admissions per 1,000 inhabitants compared to the OECD average of 15.5, 16.2 in Sweden and 12.8 in Italy) and the average duration of hospital stay (9.2 days compared to the OECD average of 7.4, 6.0 in Sweden and 7.7 in Italy); in terms of financial resources, Germany has the most important hospital network in Western Europe[19].

The **acute care hospitals** were 2,017 in the year 2012, with 501,475 beds: 601 public, 719 private non-profit and 697 private for-profit, with a split percentage split of respectively 48%, 34% and 18% of beds. In addition to acute care hospitals, 1212 structures specializing in rehabilitation exist, holding 168,968 bed places. Among these institutions, only 19% are public, 26% are private non-profit and 55% private for-profit. 18% of hospital beds are in public facilities while the other structures respectively host 16% and 66%. Next to a progressive reduction of beds for acute illnesses, the number of beds in rehabilitation and psychiatric facilities has more than doubled.

German citizens have full **freedom of choic**e of care and professional place, **with no distinction between general practitioners and medical specialists.**

This model - which **does not** include the role a of gatekeeper doctor, or a doctor who acts as a **filter for access** to specialist care - is typical of the Bismarck model, but is rapidly changing as a result of a reform approved in 2004.

Such **reform**, since **2004**, has introduced several innovations in order to strengthen local services (and to reduce the pressure on hospitals): among them is the need to encourage the enrollment of the clients to a general practitioner who in addition to playing the role of filter for access or "gatekeeper", also is responsible for the coordination of care. There is no obligation, but who does not comply is subject to reduced co-payments and waiting lists. The number of patients assisted by the "gatekeeper" or General Practitioner (GP) is growing (in 2012 to 4.6 million).

Another innovation is the overcoming of the model of care based a single physician, with the development of **medical centers of interdisciplinary care** (increased from 70 to 1,814 from 2004 to 2012).

---

19 Per la Finanza Pubblica, Commissione Tecnica. "Libro verde sulla spesa pubblica." Spendere meglio: alcune prime indicazioni (2007): 36-57.

All this is to facilitate the introduction of care pathways for some chronic diseases (with a very similar pattern to the **Chronic Care Model**), funded through a national fund and hospital-community integrated networks. The courses concern diabetes, breast cancer, ischemic heart disease, bronchial asthma and chronic obstructive pulmonary disease and have spread rapidly: in 2006 they involved 2.7 million patients, in 2012 more than 7 million, of which more than half constituted of by diabetic patients.

All these innovations would have required a strong impulse, even quantitatively, of GPs, but this was not the case. Of the 121 thousand local doctors affiliated with mutual aid, 46% are family physicians (from different backgrounds: generalists without specialization, generalists with a specialization in family medicine, internal medicine specialists, pediatricians) and 54% are specialists, with a trend increase in specialists over family physicians. This explains the **workload** found to bear by German GPs, which has no equal in other European countries: an average of 51 hours of work per week, with an average of 250 patient's contacted a week.

This is also a reason for the possibility of a nurse to be **the coordinator of care pathways** rather that the doctor..

In 1995 a new **compulsory insurance for patients with serious temporary or permanent disability**, with the same criteria of the health insurance, was introduced. Employers and employees pay 1.95% of gross monthly income (0.975% each). The 11% of the population accesses coverage through private insurance. The compulsory insurance for long-term care constitutes 8% of the financing of the health system. The facilities and services offered are graduated according to the severity of the cases (3 levels) and include financial contributions to families, ambulatory care, home and residential care. Providers are almost exclusively private, of which 36% nonprofits. In 2012 we were granted benefits and services worth 22.9 billion euro.

The **Board of Public Health** (*öffentlicher Gesundheitsdi-*

enst), present in the districts and in some large cities with the health authorities or other offices of public health, is under the control of the *Land* of competence, and is funded directly by the state. It carries out preventive activities, food safety, infectious surveillance, social care and health promotion.

Germany spends a lot on health care, but still produces a huge amount of services, with a low level of direct spending by patients. This shows that we are facing a technically **efficient** system, with short standby lists and a high user satisfaction.

But if we measure the quality of services, comparing it with that of other systems, Germany is systematically in the middle of the standings and sometimes lower. An example is that of **avoidable mortality**, where Italy and Sweden (to cite two Beveridge systems) have more positive data than Germany (and also better France, another country using the Bismarck system).

The division between **compulsory social insurance and private insurance** could lead to increasingly serious inequalities in health care.

The health care system in the **United States (US)** is predominantly private with two public assistential schemes: Medicare for retirees over age 65 and disabled people of all ages and Medicaid, instead is for the care of the poor below a certain income .

The private system is based on health **insurances** usually negotiated with the employer, which usually entail deductions directly from the worker's salary. The population not able to guarantee the payment of the annual insurance premium may be excluded from healthcare.

In order to try to counter opportunistic behavior of private insurances, **Obamacare** through the Affordable Care Act (ACA) has sought to improve access to insurance[20]. In this sense, while not presenting itself as an attempt (after Medicare and Medicaid) to make the American health care system more public,

---

20 http://healthaffairs.org/blog/2014/01/30/opting-out-of-medicaid-expansion-the-health-and-financial-impacts/ last access august 2015.

Obama's reform extension of the current private system for those who until now were excluded from it[21], thereby increasing health coverage. However, federal spending (Medicare and Medicaid) seems destined to grow again as a percentage of GDP in the next ten years[22].

In the last twenty years several attempts to redress the existing systems have taken place, especially public but also private ones, mainly in order to contain the growing expenses. Efforts have been undertaken to introduce innovations such as **"managed competition"** or **"quasi-markets"**. The latter concepts indicate the organization of an industry subject to a public intervention of regulation, thus twice underlining the critiques related to the free market and public administration. In particular, these attempts have been introduced in the Swedish and English system.

The **Canadian Health Care System** is a federal system of decentralized style, mainly financed through general taxation (Beveridge model).

21 Il sole 24ore. March 2015
22 The Economist, Don't kill Obamacare, March 2015.

2.3 The metaphor of the pendulum

As scholars of organizational sciences teach us, a **perfect** organizational model which is fine for each company, for each undertaking, for any organization **does not exist**. From time to time it is necessary to adopt the most efficient and effective approach to the needs of production or service standards to offer.

The same principle applies also and especially for more complex organizations such as those that "produce" **health**. In fact, there is no more intangible and difficulty monetizable service as the maintenance of good health, which is essential for the welfare and happiness of every individual.

It cannot be said, in fact, that a **public** health system of a state or region (model "Beveridge") is always better than a **private** health care system of a state or region (model "Bismark).

It is very likely instead, that states or regions, in order to have an efficient and effective health service must put in place a model where public and private sectors are **competing** with each other.

It is well known that health systems characterized by a private predominating model tend to migrate to the typical aspects of the public. It is also known that health systems characterized by a mainly public model, tend to migrate to typical aspects of private. This infinite **swinging** between public and private can be described as the metaphor of the pendulum. This metaphor is not exclusive of the health systems but can be extended to all the management systems of essential services such as the management of public water, energy, local mobility, waste, social services etc.

A classic example is what happened recently in the **United Kingdom (UK)** and the **United States (US)**. The UK, founder and creator of the Beveridge model, introduced private elements in its National Health Service. In contrast, the US, historical advocates of a free market health, showed a universalistic trend in access to care by realizing expansion of insurance coverage.

The system of the UK Health (National Health Service - **NHS**) was established in 1946 with the "National Health Service Act" with the purpose of guaranteeing all British citizens a centralized system inspired by the principles of solidarity and universalism for the whole health care: primary, hospital and specialised services.

In 2010, the the White Paper "Equity and Excellence: Liberating the NHS"[23] is published, becoming law in March 2012[24] with the "Health and Social Care Act 2012". Many of the changes[25] introduced by the reform affect British GPs[26]. Particularly one of the main innovations, the abolition of the Primary Care Trust (PCT) and **"Strategic Health Authorities"** (SHA) - facilities that perform similar functions to Italian regional health departments. These entities have been replaced both physically and functionally by Clinical Commissioning Group (CCG), or large consortia of family doctors (General Practitioners).

As for the **United States**, the American health care system is based mainly on the private sector, both in terms of financing, through insurance, and with regards to the supply and production of services, even with a significant public insurance component, funded by Federal and state governments[27]. Hence, the definition of the health system as based on free market. The election campaign of 1912 the Progressive candidate Theodore

---

23 Department of Health. Equity and excellence: Liberating the NHS. The Stationery Office Limited on behalf of the Controller of Her Majesty's Stationery Office: 12 July 2010

24 Health and Social Care Act 2012 chapter 7. 27th March 2012

25 Gavino Maciocco. Liberating the NHS. Svolta shock nella sanità inglese. Salute Internazionale, 02.09.2010

26 Gianfranco Damiani, Serena Carovillano, Andrea Poscia e Giulia Silvestrini. Cure primarie. Confronto shock tra UK e USA http://www.saluteinternazionale.info/2013/03/cure-primarie-confronto-shock-tra-uk-e-usa/ consultato 26 luglio 2015

Roosevelt, saw debates on the need for reform that ensures health care for all citizens[28].

Barack Obama, with the approval on March 23rd, 2010 of **health care reform**, despite having given up his idealistic goal of a Public Health Insurance, was in fact the first American President to push through a reform that aims to ensure on the one hand stabile contractual insurance conditions accessible to a greater range of citizens and on the other to contain government health spending (Medicare and Medicaid).

The shares, with the ultimate goal of improving population health outcomes, were mostly opposing the spread of **chronic diseases** (especially obesity and diabetes)[29 30].

In this context, the first steps towards a new top-level service delivery model have been taken: the **Accountable Care Organization** (ACO). This is a care model aimed exclusively to that part of health free "assistance benefiting the American population" offered by Medicare and Medicaid (both government insurance programs that the health plan offers to all citizens over sixty and dialysis patients with no age limit, and low-income groups of the populations such as children, pregnant women, disabled, indigent elderly and AIDS patients)[31 32].

---

27 World Health Report 2000. Health Systems: improving performance. WHO, Geneva, 2000. Il Rapporto è stato interamente tradotto, ed integrato per la realtà italiana, nel numero monografico di Igiene e Sanità pubblica 2001; 2:1-176

28 Gavino Maciocco. Riforma sanitaria e cure primarie negli USA. [PDF: 80 Kb]. CARE 2010; 3: 29-30

29 Armando Muzzi. La riforma sanitaria degli USA. Ig. Sanità Pubbl. 2010; 66: 147-154

30 Phillips RL, Bazemore AW. Primary care and why it matters for US health system reform. Health Aff 2010; 29: 806-810

31 Robert L. Phillips .Case Study of a Primary Care–Based Accountable Care System Approach to Medical Home Transformation. J Ambulatory Care Manage ;34(1): 67–77.

32 Managed Care – Understanding Managed Care. About.com, last access 01.05.2012.

2.4 Donald Trump and "deregulation" even in health
Angelo Barbato

First act of the Trump Presidency, in January 2017, was precisely directed at **health care** to limit the law and services obligation of the Affordable Care Act, strongly held by Barack Obama and universally recognized as Obamacare.

In first executive order of Trump, before the coming out of this book, is still not definitive since a vote of Congress is still needed. Now the US may urge a substitutive law as 20 millions of americans **risk to remain without health care.**

The lightening of rules would consent the **modification of income limitations** for the exclusion from paying premiums or allowing health care insurances to operate in more states of the country[33].

Trump has clear ideas for economic growth, simplifying procedures, rules and red tape in strategic sectors such as healthcare and energy banks. Trump is the classic example of the pendulum metaphor highlighting all his efforts towards **privatization.**

American Republicans have always pursued free-market ideas, in Ronald Reagan's words "the state is not the solution, it is the problem". Trump, at the end of January 2017, signed an executive order committing regulatory agencies to cut two rules for each new rule that will be introduced later this year.

The Congressional Budget Office, the Affordable Healthcare Act - Obamacare involves "losses of about two million full-time jobs in 2017, which would increase to about 2.5 million in 2024". As he explained by the economist Casey Mulligan in his "Side Effects and Complications: The Economic Consequences of Health-Care Reform" (University of Chicago Press, 2015), **Obamacare is a complex intrigue of incentives and subsidies,** some

---

33 http://www.ilsole24ore.com/art/mondo/2017-01-22/trump-smonta-sanita-obama-081010.shtml?uuid=AEnCuQF last access 11.02.2017

of which have a negative effect on labor and on the propensity to work harder (as the benefits diminish as income increases)[34].

Of course, as mentioned, measuring the efficiency and effectiveness of a national health system is **much more complex** than the simplistic system of public / private / mixed (organizational model - logistics) used, especially entering the field of monitoring factors of risk profiles (individual energy) and type of communication of the doctor-patient relationship.

---

34 http://www.lastampa.it/2017/02/07/esteri/sanit-banche-ed-energia-ecco-dove-trump-vuole-ridurre-le-regole-u7tyXUW1pYnlmlPOON1lzM/pagina.html-last access 11.02.2017

2.5 A new model on the horizon: the Commons of health
Bruno Corda Angelo Barbato

Various public (Beveridge) or private (Bismark) models that governed health care until now, in one way or the other, have highlighted **critical issues** related to the logical organization of the healthcare process, not integrated, especially in the main areas of management of acute illness, chronic disease, and the efficiency and effectiveness of healthcare management.

In particular, private models have revealed incongruences on the side of universality, equity and **accessibility**, while public templates have been especially weak with regards to sustainability and **efficiency**, sometimes with considerable territorial differences. Both models have expressed a significant trend increase in reported costs, due on the one hand to an evolving technology, and on the other to an ever more demanding market.

Additionally, the appearance in the health services of integrated processes of energy management (treatment of healthy patients), integrated platforms of communication (health informatics), and integrated platforms for the logistician and health transport will lead to the emergence of **smart grid digital health** which will aim to reduce the organizational entropy and the strengthening of disease prevention.

The paradigm shift: from the standby medicine to initiative medicine

From the dawn of times the patient has always turned to the man who later became a doctor, a professional trained to diagnose and treat diseases. Medicine was actually born in this way, developing on what we might call the paradigm of **standby medicine**.

The condition of being sick has always been considered

an event to intervene upon, through mobilization to solve the problem. This has developed over the centuries, the organization answers in the standby paradigm have been structured according to **emergency urgency** from the intervention of a single doctor to helicopter rescue.

The standby medicine is the **classic paradigm** of biomedical the health care model, the one on which university training of medical and health professions always rests. Academia and the medical school, over the centuries and up to now have been structured in their training mainly on the study and treatment of diseases.

The standby medicine, however, works in **urgency and emergency**, when there are no other possibilities.

Waiting too long for the course of a disease is intuitively "bad for health". Additionally, prevention, praised in recent decades has struggled in loading it into effective disease surveillance programs.

The hygienist approach in medicine, in other words considering **the holistic preventive medicine**, has began to change its overall approach to disease, introducing the concept of prevention of the disease itself by acting before it is manifested, going so far as to anticipate the different pathological states . Epidemiological studies have made a fundamental contribution to the development of anticipatory strategies.

It is understandable that the approach applied until now to ease **often been delayed**, only taking into account the moment when the patient "is sick", too often in emergency urgency, developing organizational models to contrast disease only through standby medicine, forgetting instead of acting before the disease begins its course by activating preventive medicine.

Too often, until today the patterns to contrast disease forget to include action before, through what must be a new model of health care organization and law enforcement efforts to the disease: **the medicine of initiative.**

In strategies to combat the disease a shift of paradigm becomes imperative, **from a standby medicine to initiative medicine**, also and above all because the life expectancy over the past two millennia has risen from 30 to 82.8 years in Switzerland[35] (82.7 years Italy and Japan; 82.4 years Iceland and Spain, 82.2 years France etc.) With such the increase in longevity, the ability to share long stretches one's life with a growing number of chronic diseases has also increased.

Already in a **2005** study, the American geriatric **R. Kane** pointed out that patients with one or more chronic diseases "consumed":

- 72% of the total medical visits
- 76% of all hospital admissions
- 80% of total inpatient days
- 88 % of all medical services
- 96% of all home visits.

Considering what has been said, awareness on the **initiative medicine** is growing.

In a proper application of the two paradigms, the standby cure is appropriately reflected in the medical health facilities dedicated to the urgency and emergency or high-tech care, i.e. the hospitals.

Therefore, today, in order to perform properly the **hospital** must be used to treat serious illnesses and complex diseases, acute or chronic exacerbation, with exclusive performance for emergency and urgencies, for high-tech and intensive care.

To date, the patient has **knocked** on the doctor's door.

The doctor has listened to the suffering, looking to best interpret the symptoms and therefore its condition, to proceed with most appropriate **therapy**. Consequently, the doctor and the system have improved their sensitivity and the ability to interact with the patient by orienting, guiding, helping him in the healing path, psychological even more than physical. This process has already begun and must be strengthened.

---

35 OECD. PUBLISHING. *Health at a glance 2013: OECD indicators*. OECD publishing, 2013.

With the passing of time, doctors have increasingly developed the concept that many diseases could be **preventable** and predictable even and especially through environmental and behavioral observation of individuals and communities.

While over time the hospital has been physically structuring itself in universal ways, the **area**'s facilities have been established in a disorderly and scattered manner, especially unevenly. To date, the local network is all to be seen, in many regions.

The organizational model will be more and more structured as a network, with a growing computerization of communication between doctors and patients increasingly interacting through the spread of the **Internet of things**.

The data retention will increasingly become paperless with the development of electronic health records that contain, in addition to **health data**, an **individual risk** profile of each patient.

3. The medicine initiative in the territory: prevention and chronicity

Bruno Corda Angelo Barbato Angela Meggiolaro

Already since several decades (declaration of Alma Ata on primary health care 1978) has shifted its action from health care management to the welfare of the people; consists, in practice in the professional attitude of health care providers to **prevent** the disease.

The **European action plan**[36] of the European Union, in September of 2012 determined the actions and medical objectives of the initiative with target 2020.

The **target** for the population medicine is actions by 40% of healthy individuals, 40% of healthy individuals with certain risk factors and the remaining 20% of ill individuals (of which 10% have disabilities). The prevalent health care instruments will consist of prevention and early diagnosis. The areas of competence of health professionals will be, as well as clinics, mainly epidemiological, behavioral, environmental. In addition, at the dawn of the third millennium, non-communicable diseases show a growing trend in developing countries. Therefore, it is expected that, by 2020, non-communicable diseases cause seven out of ten deaths in developing countries. Among non-communicable diseases, particular attention is devoted to cardiovascular diseases, diabetes, cancer and chronic lung diseases. The burden of these conditions applies to all countries in the world, but particularly in developing countries. Preventive strategies must take into account the increasing trend of risk factors related to these diseases[37].

Chronic Non Communicable Diseases (CNCDs) have

---

36 http://ec.europa.eu/growth/smes/promoting-entrepreneurship/action-plan/index_en.htm, last access 3.10.2015

reached a pandemic level. These diseases - which include cardio-vascular conditions (mainly heart disease and stroke), several types of cancer, chronic respiratory diseases and type 2 diabetes - affect people of all ages, nationalities and classes. About 80% of chronic disease deaths occurs in low and middle income countries. They account for 44% of premature deaths worldwide.

The **number of deaths** from these diseases is **twice** the number of deaths that result from a combination of **infectious diseases** (including HIV / AIDS, tuberculosis and malaria), **maternal** and **nutritional deficiencies** combined.

Without a concerted action, around 388 million people worldwide will die of one or more CNCDs in the next 10 years. With a taking of action, we can **prevent** millions of premature deaths among people under the age of 70.

Up to **80% of premature deaths** from heart disease, stroke and diabetes **can be prevented** with intervention strategies on chronic diseases. Yet, the prevention of disability and death from CNCDs receives little attention in the world, and even in most of the richest countries at the center of **biomedical research** on CNCDs, instead of there being prevention, there is therapy (with higher marginal gains for the multinationals).

It has been proposed **many methods for the management of chronic disease**, (*Wagner 1999 WHO World Health Organization 2002*) and many of the literature studies[38] have concluded that the most effective intervention for the treatment of chronic diseases is represented by **a multiple approach as the Chronic Care Model (CCM).**

The chronic care model (CCM) is an example of this type of approach. The model has been implemented by many organi-

---

37 Boutayeb, A. (2006). The double burden of communicable and non-communicable diseases in developing countries. Transactions of the Royal society of Tropical Medicine and Hygiene, 100(3), 191-199

38 RENDERS, Carry M., et al. Interventions to improve the management of diabetes in primary care, outpatient, and community settings. *Diabetes care*, 2001, 24.10: 1821-1833.

zations in the **United States, Canada**, the **UK** and **Sweden**[39].

This model of medical care of patients with chronic diseases was developed by Professor **Wagner** and his colleagues at the **McColl Institute for Healthcare Innovation, California**. The model proposes a series of measures to encourage improvements in the condition of the chronically ill and suggests a **"proactive" approach** between health care professionals and patients themselves, with the latter becoming an integral part of the care process.

In **Italy**, the model was adopted by the Tuscan Regional Health System in the 2008-2010 Regional Health Plan, with the objective to move from a "Standby Medicine model" for the chronic disease to an "Health Initiative model". **The new model** tries to organize a system where the need, chronic disease, turns into demand.

Hence the creation of ad hoc **paths for chronic conditions** (Assistential Diagnostic Therapeutic Protocols) such as heart failure, diabetes, hypertension, chronic obstructive pulmonary disease; therapies which require a large amount of resources from the different regional health systems. The purpose of the Chronic Care Model is to integrate this model with the hospital organization.

These are the **six directives** on which the Chronic Care Model is moving:

1. **Community resources.** To improve care for chronic patients, healthcare organizations must establish solid links with the resources of the community volunteer groups, self-help groups, self-managed senior centers.

2. **Health care organizations.** A new chronic disease management should be part of the priorities of health care providers and funders. If this does not happen it will be unlikely for innovations in care processes and even more difficult for quality to be rewarded.

---

39 WAGNER, Edward H., et al. Improving chronic illness care: translating evidence into action. *Health affairs*, 2001, 20.6: 64-78.

3. **The self-care support.** In chronic diseases the patient becomes an active protagonist of care processes. The management of these diseases can be taught to most patients.

4. **Organization of the team.** The structure of the care team (MMG, inf., Etc.) Should be changed, separating assistance for acute patients from the planned management of chronically ill patients. The MMG cures acutely ill patients, intervenes in complicated chronic cases ,. The inf. is formed to support the self care of patients and ensure the planning and conduct of follow-up of patients. The planned visit is one of the most significant aspects of the new organization.

5. **The decision support.** Adopting guidelines to provide evidence-based standards to insure optimal care of chronic patients.

6. **Information systems.** Computerized information systems have three important functions:

1) as a warning system that helps primary care team to follow the guidelines;

2) as feedback to the doctors, showing their level of performance against the indicators of chronic diseases, such as the levels of hemoglobin A1c and of lipid;

3) as disease registries to plan care of individual of patients.

4. The acute ill and first aid
Bruno Corda Angelo Barbato

The ultimate expression of standby medicine is applied in the emergency room (ER) . The latter, an essential component of any hospital is the organizational part specialized to deal 24/7 any **urgent and emergency** situation. With time, however, in the absence of a structured, organized and authoritative model that would handle not serious and non-urgent patients, the emergency room became the reference of all citizens in a situation of subjective perception of illness.

The hospital and the emergency room entered a reassuring dimension of complex and effective diagnosis and treatment of any type of emergency urgency and often less serious cases where **urgency is subjective**.

As we saw in the previous chapter, the new management paradigm has shifted from standby medicine, an effective organizational model for the acute ill, to the **medicine of initiative**, an effective proactive organizational model for the chronically ill, where the organizational asymmetry tends towards zero and takes **prevention** into account.

The two models have as common point the **acute exacerbation of a chronic disease** and in a acute/ chronic system condition and standby/ proactive initiative; certain situations that arise in the ER may also be resolved without hospitalization, through territorial care.

In some cases the episode that brings the patient to the emergency room can be considered a **"sentinel event"** due to insufficient primary care and related to the need to "relink" the sick with their care.

The emergency room is the door of the hospital for the acute patient but about a third of these accesses are classified as **non-urgent problems (about 70-75%)**. In addition, a low percentage of accesses to the emergency room **are followed by hospitalization (about 15-18%)** and even less require 24 hour observation in the hospital setting (an additional 10-12%). This data indicates a health demand profile that could be taken over by the territory.

A zonal network organization (**primary care**) with the presence of GPs available 12 hours a day or first aid points improving the organizational disorder of the system.

In lines with this hypothesis, we have recently experienced in some areas a number of innovative models **(First Aid Centres and Points)** with the same common concept: non-hospital response to urgent problems of lower gravity.

This consist of a different organization of primary care (**availability of GPs, with the possibility of relatively rapid connections with the main diagnostic services**) or First Aid Points of which results, altogether, haven not been particularly significant.

One of the most important tools used to solve or at least to ensure the primary function of the emergency room has been the **triage**, instrument through which, on the basis of standardized parameters concerning the symptoms and clinical observation of the patient, a numerical value is expressed to determine the gravity and therefore the intervention priorities. Result of such analysis are the code of severity: red, yellow, green, white, each entailing different waiting times[40]:

- **Code red**: very critical, danger of death, maximum priority, immediate access to care;
- **Code yellow**: fairly critical, presence of development of risk, can be life threatening;
- **code green**: not very critical, lack of developmental risks, deferrable performance;
- **code white**: non-critical, non-urgent patients.

---

40 http://www.salute.gov.it/portale/temi/p2_6.jsp?
lingua=italiano&id=1052&area=118%20Pronto%20Soccorso&menu=vuoto,
last access 2.09.2015

Lately there has been a trend to organize in alternative territorial structures the provision relating to situations classed as **white codes or green codes**.

Once that inside the collective imaginary of people with health needs, a present, reliable and **well organized territorial structure** will have taken shape and acquired trust, the problems of selection of input into hospitals, namely reception and emergency room will be overcome.

Hospitals, now universally established structures, are characterized by a limited organizational asymmetry while the work to be carried out in the **territory** is much larger for the high proportion of **organizational asymmetry** to break down.

Surely in the evolution of systems, reducing the organizational asymmetry in the territory also automatically it **improves the hospital's organizational asymmetry**.

On the hospital side, the control of inflows through the door of the emergency room is the paradigm of the **Emergency Department** as a safety valve for hospital inefficiencies, towards the modern vision of Emergency itself in a highly interconnected organic system.

The **main directives** for this objective are:

1) the **diversification** of the flows in the emergency department between patients with high or low need of care. Example of this diversification is the creation of the surgery "minor codes" for those patients with almost always solvable problems with limited engagement of clinical and instrumental resources, to order to contain excessive waiting time and stay in the emergency department. In addition, the "fast track" programs must also be integrated to allow to deal safely and relatively rapidly (24-48 h) with clinical situations that do not require an immediate solution. Diversification is a choice consistent with the option of an offer depending on the extent of need: to this end, the health services are committed to ensuring the full use of the procedures described above, including adapting staffing of medical personnel and nursing emergency-urgency;

2) a different management of **intra-hospital flows**. The current organization has two main characteristics:

a) a **"pulsed" flow** of discharges (once a day) that determines a host unavailability of shelters for large part of the day;

b) a commission of the chosen hospitalizations with those of urgency in the same spaces. The reorganization of hospitals based on care of different intensity must provide for the separation of the two lines so that the shelters in one area shall not interfere negatively on the functionality of the other. Moreover, the flow of the discharges must be based on greater continuity in the 24 hours through, for example, the creation of specific structures for the expectation of discharge (**discharge room**) and a better organization of transport services;

3) **diagnostic imaging** must be part of the technological equipment at least in high influx ERs. Excessive lengths of stay in the Emergency Department are often attributable to merge into a single diagnostic service inquiries from several parts of the health system (hospital, community, DEA);

4) the creation of a modern **computerized link** across the various segments of the routes in emergency-urgency (phone line, PS, hospitalization areas, primary care). A good recording/reporting of data makes care work safer and more efficient, allowing critical analysis and comparison of and between the various involved structures.

These important technical and organizational aspects should not relegate to a secondary plane the problem of **reception**, meaning the ability to create for the patient and his family a place and an atmosphere in which you can **hold and manage the inevitable anxieties**. First of all, the old idea that a citizen may appeal to the emergency department without any plausible reason must be finally overcome. The lack of effective alternatives elsewhere or a situation perceived as subjective urgency does constitute, in the current cultural landscape, reasons that can not be treated as invalid.

Secondly, creating a **good reception** implies adopting

structural measures to improve the standby and working environments, guaranteeing privacy, good triage, managing needs
during waiting... Such needs may not only be strictly clinical. In
other words, patients should be "accompanied" during their time
in the emergency room until the time of discharge or admission
which must take place in clear and understandable terms.

Ultimate goal is to make the hard impact with the emergency room a moment of reassurance for citizens and an encour-
agement of confidence for the next path in the system.

5. Prevention

5.1 Introduction
Bruno Corda, Angelo Barbato

Rethinking **access to health services** by the citizens as a matter of fairness requires to take into account demographic, epidemiological, social and economic trends across different territories.

Zero Disease is a strategy that aims to boost prevention and preventive medicine with a systemic vision that emphasizes the causes and the risk factors related to the environment illness, zero.

It is opposed to the fragmented vision of a **single case** disease that often manifests itself through an emergency urgent condition.

In the study of disease distribution, **two criteria** are adopted, placing the observational process in different timeframes.

The **first criterion** limits the observation only to events that are generated from scratch during a specified period of time (usually a year) in a population in which they had not come forward before and that, therefore considered "new" cases.

This measure takes the name of **incidence.**

The **second criterion** consists in the enumeration of the events present at a given time in a defined population. This constitutes a measure which is called of **predominance**, as present in a certain instant in time (photography).

The goal of **primary prevention** is to counter the occurrence of new cases of disease. Therefore, a primary prevention intervention produces a decrease in the incidence rate of the disease to which it is addressed: the higher the taking of action, the more the incidence is reduced.

To achieve the reduction of the incidence of the disease in the population it is necessary to reduce the **individual risk**; this can be reduced to zero if you can permanently remove the cause of the disease or prevent it from continuing to act on the population.

The population must be aware of the application of healthy **lifestyles** through interventions of education and health promotion.

The general measures of health protection and safety of workers in the **workplace** fall under the zero disease strategy.

Effective tools for primary prevention of infectious diseases are surveillance, information and health education, and vaccinations.

The **surveillance** of infectious diseases is based on accurate vigilance of these pathologies.

Health is increasingly involved in assessing the aspects associated with **environmental** issues. Not surprisingly, the EU Action Plan on Environment and Health 2004 - 2010 and the European health strategy called "Together for Health - A Strategic Approach for the EU 2008-2013", considers it essential to implement the system of knowledge locally, concerning the health-environment relationship.

These actions entail the improvement of **air** quality, **water** and **soil**, **food safety**, **noise reduction**, control of risks linked to **electromagnetic fields** and protection from **ionizing radiation**.

Secondary prevention is aimed at the discovery and healing of cases of illness before they manifest clinically and in any case as soon as possible. The advantage of early diagnosis in the preclinical phase is that therapy will give a better chance of definitive cure. Consequently, a well conducted secondary prevention intervention will determine a disability or reduction in mortality, of which the amount of significance will depend on the efficacy of the intervention itself. It may also produce a decrease in the prevalence of those diseases of gradually discovered cases and immediately subjected to care, thereby quickly healing, while cases diagnosed in advanced clinical stage have a long course before reaching healing or death. Instead, secondary prevention has no effect of reduction on the incidence. In fact, unlike primary prevention, it does not remove the causes of a disease and, consequently, does not avoid the occurrence of new cases.

The aging trend of the population, with the consequent increase in the relevance of **chronic diseases**, exposes to the system the need to cope with the change of welfare demand through a response to the complex needs characterized by a strong socio-health integration.

The analysis of the health profile highlights increases in prevalence of some chronic diseases of great importance:

- **diabetes** - patients being treated with anti-diabetic drugs, a fifth of whom treated with insulin;
- **hypertension** - patients taking antihypertensive drugs;
- **acute myocardial infarctions (AMI)**;
- **brain stroke**;
- elderly over sixty with **heart failure**;
- Patients over 65 with **chronic obstructive pulmonary disease (COPD)**.

With regards to comorbidities, it is estimated that seniors with at least **three chronic illnesses** are about 9% of over sixty-five year olds.

It is consequently crucial to **rethink organizational models** aiming to develop integrated care contained in an organic context of roles and functions, thereby removing the obstacles to professionals' integration. In this view, the "capacity" of the system to take charge of the promotion of health through appropriate primary prevention initiatives assumes a particular value. Such is the adoption of healthy lifestyles, particularly the exercise of physical activity and the uptaking of good eating habits, which must however be seen not only as a prevention tool but also as indispensable aid to the therapies in the management of disease in the event of its outbreak.

In the philosophy of adoption of the new model, secondary prevention and screening must be integrated with the primary role during early diagnosis of many chronic diseases. This new tool will contain the **individual risk profile** contained in the personalized health document, available and updated.

5.2 The determinants of health
Bruno Corda, Angelo Barbato, Angela Meggiolaro

The determinants of health are the factors that **influence** (change in frequency and in characters of a disease) in a positive or negative state of health of an individual and - more broadly - of a community or population.

Monofactorial etiology diseases, in which not only a single cause is at stake, is also referred to as "monofactorial etiology" or "mono-factorial diseases." These diseases are generated by such a strong cause as to be capable by itself, to cause all the events that lead to the appearance of the disease.

In **multifactorial etiology** diseases, the sickness is the result of a highly complex interaction of several factors (external or internal to the body), which act simultaneously or in succession on the organism, in synergism or antagonism with each other. These diseases are called "multi-factorial" or "multifactorial etiology".

The cause (**etiology**) of a disease can be any factor, element, circumstance which gives origin to an effect (disease) or to a sequence of events that result in the effect.

In epidemiology, the **risk** represents the probability for an individual or a population, that an event (typically the disease) will occur at a given time or in a given period of time.

Instead, with the term **"determinant"** the concept of cause as "factor capable of increasing the probability" of the disease is introduced. The concept of determinant is anyway closely related to 'risk' as it refers to all the factors that are able to influence the appearance or development of a disease, while not being considered "cause" of the disease in the strict sense.

The **primary determinants** are represented by factors whose variation exerts a greater effect in the genesis of the disease. In other words, they are of fundamental importance for the appearance of the disease.

The **secondary determinants** are represented by factors whose variation exerts a smaller effect in the genesis of the disease. In other words, they are neither essential nor crucial for the appearance of the disease. In many cases they represent the so-called "predisposing" or "favoring" factors. Secondary determinants can be divided into intrinsic (or endogenous, i.e. internal to their host) and extrinsic (or exogenous)[41].

The **positive determinants** are those factors that reduce the risk of disease in the individual or in the community. Consider, for example, proper nutrition, the practice of a sport, reading, or earning an adequate income, etc.

Negative determinants are all those factors which favour the risk of diseases.

For example, a sedentary lifestyle, smoking or alcohol abuse, but also the loss of a job, or a unsuitable accommodation. The study of the determinants of health and illness allows you to process multiple interventions (Primary health-care) in order to reduce the incidence of the disease while increasing the well-being perceived by the person and the community[42].

Interventions in these fields are not exclusive domain of the health services, but can involve **every sector** of society.

Accredited international studies have performed a quantitative estimation of some elements on the longevity of the community, used as indirect indicator of well-being: the socio-economic factors and **lifestyles** contribute by **40-50%**; the status and conditions of the **environment** by **20-30%**; **genetic inheritance** by another **20-30%**, and health services by **10-15%**[43].

41
http://www.unipegaso.it/materiali/Scienze/annoII/Igiene_Giella/ModI/Lezione_I.pdf, last access 31.10.2015
42 Gavino Macciocco http://www.saluteinternazionale.info/2009/01/i-determinanti-della-salute-una-nuova-originale-cornice-concettuale/ consultato 31.10.2015
43 https://it.wikipedia.org/wiki/Determinanti_della_salute last access 4.10.2015

There are **conceptual models** that put out one factor over another, when a hierarchy of values among the various elements is established.

According to the **first model**[44], people's health it would be conditioned by 50% from their behavior and their lifestyles. Other determinants are given much less importance: environmental factors (20%), genetic factors (20%), health care (10%). This is a model that focuses on the role of the of people's lifestyles and reflects the emphasis that in the United States is placed in individual responsibility in health and disease.

The **second model**, according to the schools of public health in northern Europe, the factors affecting the health status are expressed in a series of concentric layers, each corresponding to different levels of influence. At the center is the individual, with its biological characteristics: gender, age, genetic inheritance: these health determinants which are not editable. The modifiable determinants, those that are likely to be corrected and processed, move from the inner layers to the outermost: individual lifestyles, social and community networks, the living and working environment, the political environment, social, economic, cultural levels and the psychological structure.

The distinction between models of health determinants based on their **hierarchical values**, although representing an interesting academic argument is not provided in the setting of this story due to the complication of distinguishing between determinants influenced directly from adequate health and independent interventions. Moreover, the weight of a determinant with respect to another has a relative and personalized value.

This is why it becomes important to build the health identikit of the patient, centered on its **risk profile** and **maintenance program**.

The patient wants to feel **protected**, subsequently advised, informed, reassured and, when necessary, treated. But all

---

44 NATIONAL CENTER FOR HEALTH STATISTICS, et al. US Centers for Disease Control and Prevention. *Multiple Cause of Death*, 1999, 2013.

this he expects from a professional or better from a highly competent, sensitive and authoritative professional setting. Medicine has evolved, you work more and more as a team, with sophisticated diagnostic tools.

The **relationship between doctor and patient** is always the basic prerequisite for the establishment of trust essential for an effective health intervention and its effect over time. In order for this to happen, the patient appeals to a therapist who, if in possession of a correct empathetic attitude, allows the fundamental relationship of trust. The latter is defined by Carl Rogers as that attitude needed to create a climate of security useful to bring out the individual resources. "What I am is enough, if only I can be so". The statement perfectly sums up the author's thought. And here is where the therapist, doctor or psychologist, or who it may be; he who has the task to advise, guide and satisfy the process of adaptation and growth of the individual who gives his trust, thereby starting the healing process. Here appears to its full extent the concept of empathy and collaboration, requirements in Rifkin's innovative thinking revolution to guarantee, in the environmental vision, survival.

This applies to **any organizational context**, in particular for what interests us: the health in its broadest and modern sense!

Obviously, this innovative approach finds applied problems in different regions of the world, especially in the realization of the right balance between **Holistic medicine**, already supported by empirical indicators, and **traditional medicine**, closely related to indicators based on scientific evidence. These two interpretations of medical science have often created conflicting professional situations, leaving large areas of intervention to economic and political, private and public power groups.

5.3 The determinants of social and economic integration and social welfare

Angelo Barbato, Angela Meggiolaro

Several studies have documented the existence of a significant predictive ability of health or mortality, based on **socio-economic** deprivation indices measured at the block level or micro-areas of census, net of compositional effects[45].

It is well known that within a city or a country we are districts of high internal homogeneity - i.e. places of life uniformly deprived, exposed to **environmental toxicity** or **unhealthy lifestyles** - of which structural features may impact to varying degrees on the state of its people's health.

Income **poverty** provides, at best, an incomplete explanation of the differences in mortality between countries or between subgroups within a country. In addition, it is well known that among the rich countries there is only a weak correlation between GDP per capita and life expectancy. Greece, p. e.g., with a GDP at constant purchasing power of just over $ 17,000, has a life expectancy of 78.1 years life; the US, with a GDP of over $ 34,000, has a life expectancy of 76.9 years. Costa Rica and Cuba stand out as countries with a GDP of less than $ 10,000 but with a life expectancy of 77.9 and 76.5 years of life.

Inequalities in health between and within states are **reducible**. There is no real biological reason why life expectancy is 48 years longer in Japan than in Sierra Leone or 20 years shorter among Australian Aborigines and Torres Strait Islanders than other Australians. Reducing these social inequalities in health, therefore addressing human needs, is a matter of social justice[46].

The **determinants** to be monitored are: culture, under-

---

45 PICKETT, Kate E.; PEARL, Michelle. Multilevel analyses of neighbourhood socioeconomic context and health outcomes: a critical review. *Journal of epidemiology and community health*, 2001, 55.2: 111-122.

stood in a broad sense, socioeconomic status (factors which in turn will influence the behaviors and lifestyles) and the environment, understood as ecosystem. To these determinants on health and social welfare must then be added the individual genetic heritage and, finally, the availability and access to "universal" health care *(Figure 1)*[47].

Figure 1: Determinants of health well-being. (Adapted from: Department of Social Health Works Section I eco-socio-economic determinants of health by: G. Domenighetti, J. Quaglia, L. Inderwildi Bonivento Bellinzona, November 2000)

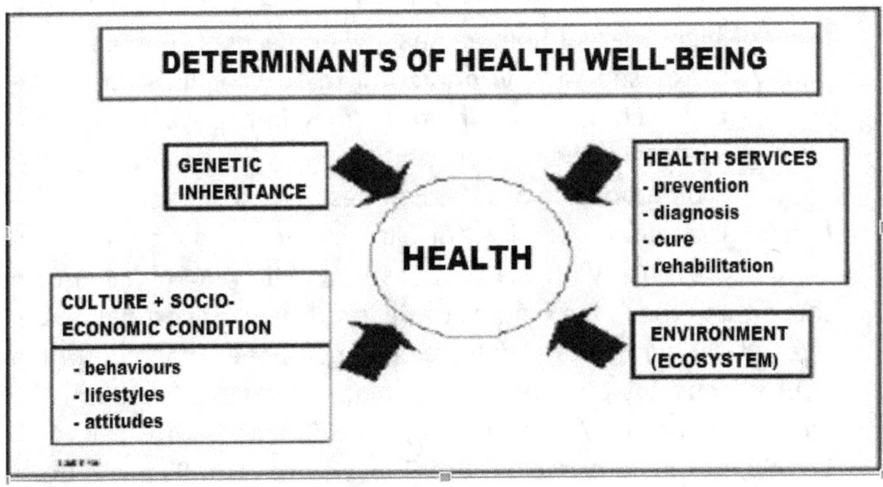

Disease can affect a person's social position, compromising his chances of employment and reducing his income; as well as, at the community level, certain epidemic diseases (e.g. AIDS in Africa), which can produce serious damage on the functioning of social, economic and political institutions. In the Rio Political Declaration on Social Determinants of 2011 (Ministry of Health Rio Declaration on Social Health Determinants, Rio de Janeiro,

---

46 Di Michael Marmot - Lancet 2005; 365: 1099–104 Determinanti sociali delle disuguaglianze nella salute

47 Gavino Macciocco Salute Internazionale 2009. I determinanti della salute. Una nuova, originale cornice concettuale

76

Brazil, October 21st, 2011) there is a commitment to adopt appropriate health measures able to act transversally and to develop policies aimed at promoting global health but with special attention to the vulnerable population. **Social Determinants** thus enter with full rights in the concept of health promotion, holding stand even in the idea of "health" at political, social, personal level, in addition to in the daily health work. Recognition of the "political" importance of health determinants, results in fact in a basic concept in the epidemiology.

Integrating social welfare and the promotion of synergy is the lever for "change" aimed at a structural renewal of the productive and social system as a whole.

"The good living" is therefore configured as an identity connected to an expanded vision of development, understood as resulting from the convergence, **integration** and inter-sectoral policies for the development of human resources, job security, education , the environment, health and the promotion of healthy lifestyles.

It is important to identify clear **priorities:**

• to focus on innovative organizational models, on **integrating socio-territorial** health care, for the extension of the potential offer in currently lacking areas or not provided for, and to give greater effect to the welfare integrated responses with expanded social interventions (to housing, mobility, leisure, etc.);

• define the central role of assistance to the **dependent person** receiving care and family support, to cope with the social effects of the aging population and increase coverage provided by the various forms of intervention;

• promote the integration of **immigrants**, to foster trust in the institutions.

5.4 Lifestyles

Angelo Barbato, Angela Meggiolaro

Lifestyle is a **way of living** based on identifiable patterns of behavior determined by the interaction between personal characteristics of an individual and social, socio-economic and environmental conditions[48].

These patterns of **behavior** are not fixed, but subject to change. Individual lifestyles, characterized by identifiable patterns of behavior, can have a profound effect on the health of the individual and the community. Health is maintained and conquered supporting the individual to make lifestyle changes, however, the action must be geared to the social and cultural conditions that help produce and maintain these patterns of behavior.

There is no "optimal" lifestyle, prescribable universally. Culture, income, family structure, age, physical ability, work environment affect the most appropriate lifestyle[49].

According to the 2002 report of the **World Health Organization**, there are some risk factors that can actually influence and negatively affect the length of a man's life. Following, the data related to the **loss of years** due to risk factors in industrialized countries is presented:

- 12.2 Nicotine addiction
- 10.9 Hypertension
- 9.2 Alcohol
- 7.6 Hypercholesterolemia
- 7.4 Overweight

48
http://www.who.int/healthpromotion/conferences/previous/ottawa/en/,last access 31.10.2015
49
http://apps.who.int/iris/bitstream/10665/64546/1/WHO_HPR_HEP_98.1.pdf?ua=1 , last access 02.09.2015

- 3.9 Reduced consumption of fruits and vegetables
- 3.3 Sedentary
- 1.8 illicit substances

It should be noted that this research takes into account one factor at a time, thus not correlating it to others, so their simultaneous effect must be considered as a sum of values, thus aggravating the situation of returnees in multiple categories[50].

---

50 https://it.wikipedia.org/wiki/Stile_di_vita, last access 02.09.2015

5.5 Physical activity
Roberto del Gaudio

Based on an idea of heath development, which finds its maximum evolution in the paradigm of Zero Zone, let us first find out what health is, not only observing it from a medical scientific point of view, but from optic of **sport**. Health must be understood as the maximum expression of the body's functionality, in all its aspects: good condition of the internal organs of the body, joint mobility, muscle tone and flexibility as well as a psychological balance of the individual.

Let us analyze in a few lines such conditions:

- **Physical Health** in the strict sense, is obtained from a prior physical fitness;

- **Mobility** is achieved with a performance of gentle exercise by activating all the joints of the body;

- **Firmness** through physical exercises that engage the body in resistances, through both free-body exercises as with weights or using water as a medium;

- **Flexibility** is reached and cultivated with an ongoing commitment from a type of relaxed stretching to the stretching of the muscles;

- **Mental health**, that is a mental stability, also derives from sport activity calibrated on the individual person.

A **non-agonist** sportsman will seek in the long-term, to maintain a satisfactory state of health as well as an appropriate overall fitness condition.

The body already ages independently, if then we add **non-appropriate physical activity** and not related to the quality of life applied to the individual, the effects would be disastrous. Due to what?

Due to an unbalancing in our mental and physical, energetic and health **equilibrium.**

The concept of Health must not be separated from that of personal exercise (fitness); only an effective exercise appropriate for the individual will lead to the achievement of the most desired and pursued effect: **physical Wellness** (feeling good and being trained in mental and physical balance with yourself).

In turn, Wellness produces, as effect and continuous research, **Anti Aging**, which represents maintenance and potential optimization of wellness' objective.

The **Fitness** terminology is used to indicate the physical activity needed to achieve the goal of the shape, ie the individual's physical fitness.

What is the difference with sport?

The latter is the execution of motor activities that have as their purpose the **training** of the body, in addition to being a means for obtaining the physical shape (Fitness).

Among the so-called "**gym sports**", many gyms have divided the world of fitness as follows:

CARDIOVASCULAR CAPACITY:

• **step**: entailing a series of dynamic exercises of stepping up and down from the platform following the rhythm punctuated by the music;

• **spinning**: aerobic activity with the use of a bike, it is possible to combine this discipline with the use of small weights for the execution of exercises for the upper body;

• **zumba**: essentially dance lessons with cardio activity with alternating high and low intensity Latin dances and more. Variants may be the Aqua Zumba, then in the pool or even the Zumba Step, a combination of dances by the use of the characteristic step platform of this sport;

• **hidrobike**: spinning in the water, for an even more intense training than the Earth's version;

MUSCULAR STRETCHING:

• **stretching**: a series of muscular stretching exercises, used to prevent muscle and tendon injuries, with the improvement of the articular range of improvement;

- **yoga**: ascetic and meditative practices, similar to martial arts for the balance the self, like Tai Chi Chuan;

TONING:

- **Pump**: resistance activity that activates the red fibers of the muscles through their exercises of Bodybuilding but with very small loads;
- **TRX**: endurance activities through the use of circuits in which ropes with slings are used to perform exercises for all muscle groups. In this way the weight of the body is exploited to counter resistance;
- **buttocks, legs and abdominals**, therefore a series of exercises aimed at training these muscle areas;
- **Upper Training**: general gymnastics exclusively for the upper body
- **circuit training** with Body Building machines: circuits without pause or nearly so, through the use of machinery and their exercises particular of the Physical Culture;
- **Aquafitness**: water gymnastics using water resistance to train the body. With this activity it is possible to combine the use of small weights for a more invigorating workout, etc.;

Bodybuilding is an approach to training with opposition resistance that today is unmatched in the sportiv world. With this exercise you train your body to get stronger, toned, activator of all muscle areas, you will come to obtain an increase in resting metabolic rate, training the heart, and you can reach a significant fat loss with appropriate training systems.

Bosu is the use of a half sphere as an activator of proprioception. By using this tool as a basis, we can perform countless bodyweight exercises, using the balance of the body under stress. It is also possible to include isometric movements.

Dance with all its specialties: modern, hip hop, Latin American dances are examples of physical activity that appeals more to the individual.

Martial arts, like **swimming**, are regarded as comprehensive sports thanks to their activation of all the muscles of the body, and because the practitioner goes into the integrative study of Eastern philosophies also marking internal mental energy discoveries.

Many sports centers offer a "**club package**", which includes different activities that the gym has to offer. The basic idea is to try to attract more people taking advantage of the wide range of specialties. This formula, however, often leads more towards the psychological satisfaction of the client rather than to the physical shape. Varying sports not because one was drafted a personalized weekly activity program with which one takes advantage of the various activities for specific objectives, but for marketing reasons against boredom. In doing so one does not reach "fitness" through perseverance and dedication.

The term **wellness** is an extension and evolution of the concept of fitness: it refers to a philosophy of life that puts the well-being of the person at the center offering sports activities, regeneration practices as well as mental training combined with proper nutrition . Wellness encourages a state of well-being and mental and physical balance[51].

Hot springs (even spas or Spa) are public or private facilities for the administration of hydrotherapy. Since the sixteenth century, the word spa, from the Belgian town Spa, known since the fourteenth century for its mineral waters, became the term par excellence for the hot springs, first in English and then in other languages. The term is interpreted by some in retrospect as an acronym for Latin expressions such as *salus per aquam* or *sanare per aquam*, cases in which it can be found written in uppercase (SPA)[52].

The wellness and spa are a set of practices, not only sportive, but also of relative relax, inducing a state of well-being and relaxation of both the body as of the **mind.**

The SPA, however, produces a sense of "momentary health", as indeed any massage can make only a **very short pe-**

---

51 https://it.wikipedia.org/wiki/Wellness , last access 06.10.2015
52 https://it.wikipedia.org/wiki/Terme ,last access 06.10.2015

riod of relaxation to ensure that the person feels good with himself. So what are we dealing with? Orientation to Wellness is an effect and not a means. All that is currently intended for Wellness is actually an integration of a set of multiple FITNESS activities (staying in shape). Let me explain: you have to use the world of sport in its interrelationship with all the factors that are part of it (programmed and personalized physical activity, proper nutrition, supplementation if needed, adequate recovery between workouts and adequate sleep based on the needs of the individual); everything is Fitness.

This physical form will bring along the real "wellness" effect: a state of well-being that will not fade within a few hours, but if protracted, slowly will turn into a **lifestyle** for the longevity of the individual.

What are the combinations of **health and fitness**? Essentially 4:

1) To be healthy but with poor physical fitness: in this case a slow and progressive approach to sport is the way forward;

2) To not be healthy, and not in shape: medical interventions with soft physical activity is the most suitable process for this purpose;

3) To be healthy and in good shape: the top of the cases that may arise. In this condition it is necessary to focus essentially on sports goals, both anaerobic and aerobic;

4) To not be healthy, but quite trained: this is referring to athletes who have always practiced sports in which they need: power, stretching, attention in the rest.

It is therefore important to practice regular **physical activity**[53] by finding a temporal space. Even little time available, if well designed, will give vitality and energy not only to the body but also to the psyche.

The concept of **Energy**, basic paradigm of Zero Zone,

---

53 La scienza dell'esercizio resa semplice di Brian Johnston Sandro Ciccarelli editore

when marked to medicine, is considered the fundamental condition for physical well-being. Without energy we can not react to performing any form of mental fatigue when this is arises.

The second fundamental paradigm is **Communication,** that in physical activity takes place in a horizontally with teammate or training companions and in a vertical manner with the coach.

The third paradigm is the **Logistics,** which in relation to the fitness world is the place where you actually work out. The gym is a suitable place where train with or without a personal trainer and workout plans[54], or through applications created for fitness.

Health and physical activities are always integrated[55]. The Latin phrase **Mens sana in corpore sano** (literally: Healthy mind in a healthy body) is accredited to Juvenal (Satires, X, 356)[56]. In modern usage it means that for having healthy mental faculties, you have to have health even for the body by virtue of psychophysical unity[57].

---

54 https://it.pinterest.com/explore/programmi-di-fitness-899993928408/, last access 5.10. 2015

55 https://www.hardgainer.com, last access 5.10. 2015

56 https://it.wikipedia.org/wiki/Mens_sana_in_corpore_sano, last access 5.10. 2015

57 Sentenze, motti, proverbi latini brevemente illustrati, appendice al Vocabolario della Lingua Latina Campanini-Carboni, Paravia, Torino, 1993, p. 50.

5.6 The prevention of chronic degenerative diseases through nutrition

Antonina Fazio

The need of a worldwide adoption, at regional and national levels, of the **prevention** and control of chronic illnesses, particularly cardiovascular diseases, diabetes and cancer, has been recognized as an urgent policy prerogative, from the document of the general assembly of the United Nations.

In this regard, the work plan led by the WHO, allowed to document the mortality trend for chronic diseases and the prevalence of certain risk factors associated with them, in respect of each member country. The data were published in July 2014, in the report "Noncommunicable Diseases - Country Profiles 2014" which shows that, in Western countries, cancer mortality is around 30%, while **mortality** from cardiovascular causes ranges between 28 % and 40%. The prevalence of these diseases is constantly increasing, since, from the economic point of view, results in progressive unsustainability in health, increase of morbidity and thus reduced productivity at the enterprise level and in purely human terms , an indecipherable cost of suffering.

Any intervention aimed at primary prevention of chronic degenerative diseases requires the control of associated risk factors. In this sense the most recent scientific evidence shows clearly that certain dietary patterns can be an effective means of reducing all metabolic risk factors s**uch as type 2 diabetes, dyslipidemia, hypertension** and **obesity**, both related to cancer and to cardiovascular disease.

Obesity[58], as well as in the case of a normal weight per-

---

58 defined by a BMI> 30 kg / m2. The body mass index (abbreviated or BMI, body mass index English) is a biometric data, expressed as a ratio between weight and square of the height of an individual.It is used as a form of the weight status indicator.

son, abdominal obesity[59], or a high ratio waist circumference / hip circumference (WHratio), certainly represent a risk factor, especially for cardiovascular diseases and diabetes type 2, as well as for many forms of cancer, mainly for breast cancer in postmenopausal and colon-rectal cancer.

The pathophysiological mechanism by which obesity is able to promote chronic degenerative diseases is the fact that obesity is associated with:

• altered levels of **adipokines**: the adipose tissue has not only the excess energy storage function ; is also an endocrine organ, that is capable of producing such adipokines hormones, including leptin and adiponectin, regulators of various biological functions which also influence tumor growth and immune function;

• **chronic state of inflammation**: the expansion of adipose tissue (particularly in the abdominal seat) and hypertrophy of the fat cells, are the result of an excess of calorie intake, causing an infiltration of macrophages. Once activated, these contribute, together with the fat cells, to the secretion of pro-inflammatory, mutagenic, anti-apoptotic and pro angiogenic adipokines. They therefore, in summary, promote tumor growth, in addition to the secretion of inflammatory cytokines including IL-6 and TNFalpha, which causes local and systemic inflammation; becomes chronic and can consequently contribute to carcinogenesis, atherosclerosis and to other chronic degenerative processes;

• high **insulin** levels: in cases of abdominal obesity (or just overweight), you establish an inflammatory state, which together with the reduction of the adiponectin hormone, produced by the fat tissue, is associated primarily with insulin resistance, mediated by the same adipokines, followed by a compensatory hyperinsulinemia with increased hepatic glucose production and alterations in lipoprotein profile or hypertriglyceridemia, increased LDL and decreased fraction of so-called "good" cholesterol or

---

59 Abdomen circumference above a determined threshold value.

HDL (which stands for High Density Lipoprotein). This certainly is a risk factor for type 2 diabetes, hypertension and cardiovascular diseases. Being insulin a hormone that stimulates itself mitogenesis, (i.e. growth in several tissues including tumoral tissues, presenting insulin receptors type A) and responsible for the increase in blood levels and bioavailability of fundamental factors for tumor growth, such as IGF-I and estrogen, hyperinsulinemia is also associated with increased cancer risk;

- alteration of **intestinal flora**: the intestinal dysbiosis, induced by diet, is associated with an increased risk not only of obesity, including cardiovascular disease, cancer, but also of allergies and autoimmune diseases;

- increase in cellular **metabolic activity,** which can result in DNA damage through the overproduction of oxygen compounds at high oxidant activity, produced during metabolism (ROS)[60].

Maintaining a healthy weight, with a BMI <25kg/m^2 and especially to **maintain the waist**, is therefore the first goal to also prevent cancer. Even more so for those who are already fighting cancer, this is important to facilitate the action of eventual chemotherapy and to improve the prognosis. This highlights how important it is strongly oppose the current rising incidence of obesity in children, as the obese child often evolves into an obese adult.

But are there **specific foods and/or beverages**, which can directly affect weight gain?

The results obtained from one of the large prospective studies, which investigated, subjecting hundreds of thousands of normal weight subjects in alimentary questionnaires, the relationship between the weight increase and the assumption of different diet components, regardless of other lifestyle factors, show that **the gradual gain of weight**, dose-dependent, is strongly associated with the consumption of: **french fries, potatoes** and **sugary drinks** mainly, followed by **red meat** and **pre-**

---

60 Reactive Oxygen Species http://www.ncbi.nlm.nih.gov/pubmed/11076791, last access 15 .10. 2015

served meats, refined flour, sweets and desserts, "trans" fats.

Instead, **counteracting** weight gain are **vegetables, whole grains, fresh and dried fruit, yogurt.** The outcome of this study confirms that consumption of high-glycemic foods, such as potatoes and precisely refined flour (in particular 0 and 00) favors (as well as the consumption of processed foods high in sugar, fat and added salt) weight gain. This because these are foods that quickly and in greater quantity raise blood sugar levels, causing a consequent greater insulin response, which promptly lowers the concentration of glucose in the blood and stimulates the hunger signal, and with it, a probable increase in calories consumed.

In the perspective of **prevention,** therefore, the consumption of cereals and wholemeal flour is desirable, as proven inter alia by several epidemiological studies, which have shown the protective effect against chronic-degenerative diseases; not only for the action modulating on blood glucose levels, but also for that **fraction of non-starchy polysaccharide fiber.** It is from the latter that refined flours are instead depleted, thereby becoming non degradable by enzymes of our intestine, and which is metabolized by specific colonies present in our intestinal flora, that colonizes it.

From the microbial fermentation of whole grain fiber (such as legumes and vegetables), one of the metabolites produced are **short-chain fatty acids** (SCFAs)[61] from polysaccharide molecules, such as arabinoxylans and beta glucans, the proportion of which depends not only on fermentable substrate and therefore the amount of fiber from cereal ingested, but also by the microbial composition. . This is due to the fact that only a few species are able to produce SCFAs and only at determined intestinal pH values.

Among SCFAs, **butyrate** plays an important role in the intestinal mucosa, which is a nutrient medium, capable of influencing gene expression of the epithelial cells of the colon, reducing

---

61 Short Chain Fat Acids (mainly acetate, propionate and butyrate)

inflammation and fighting the process of carcinogenesis, as shown by experiments in vitro.

Besides the SCFAs that pass into the bloodstream, although in micromolar concentrations, also play a beneficial metabolic role, being able to act at the adipose tissue level, which interferes with the production of adipokines hormones and thus improves glucose homeostasis and insulin sensitivity.

The consumption of whole grains also increases the intestinal colonization of **bifidobacteria**, able to modulate the inflammation also outside of the colon and to counteract the growth of those intestinal microbes that promote obesity.

A cohort study also showed that the consumption of **whole grains** reduces the risk of visceral adiposity.

Even a modest calorie restriction can promote the reduction of the growth of **harmful microbes** or anyway those associated with obesity, and the increase of beneficial ones, which thus promote weight loss.

The reduction in calorie intake, therefore, contrasts certainly the chance of obesity. More and more experimental data, conducted in several animal models, also shows that **calorie restriction**, associated with adequate nutrition, providing proper intake of vitamins and minerals, increases longevity and slows aging. Even more importantly, it protects against type 2 diabetes, cardiovascular disease, hypertension, inflammation and metabolic risk factors associated with cancer.

Experiments in animal models, and in the genetic and pharmacological field, also indicate that the **reduction of the availability of aminoacids and calories** in the diet significantly increases the lifetime and reduces the risk of disease. This results in the cell, in a modulation of the molecular pathway sensitive to the availability of nutrients (PI3K/AKT and mTOR).

In parallel, studies on humans suggest that a moderate and sustained **calorie restriction** produces trends of metabolic adaptations such as reducing total cholesterol, LDL, fasting glucose, C-reactive protein and high blood pressure. Thereby decreasing the risk of type 2 diabetes, abdominal obesity, hypertension, lipid disorders, inflammation, cancer and cardiovascular diseases.

This is on the condition that calorie restriction also provides adequately quality and quantity of nutrients's intake. This suggests, in summary, that the calorie intake and the quality of the diet can ensure that aging is not inevitably a condition linked to these pathologies. The scientific data collected in this area show that the beneficial effects on metabolic risk factors are related, first of all, to the assumed kind of nutrients, or the **quality of the diet**.

This is confirmed by the data on the reduction of risk factors such as blood pressure, blood lipids and blood sugar in people with **vegan diet**, without calorie restriction. Therefore calorie restriction alone is not a prerogative of sufficient preventive effect.

In fact, the dietary pattern emerged from the beneficial effects of calorie restrictions in humans has provided for the **elimination of high-glycemic foods** such as refined carbohydrates, potatoes, white rice, enriched foods of sucrose and/or fructose, rich in processed foods salt, trans fatty acids, and the corresponding increase in the intake of a wide variety of vegetables, **low-glycemic** fruits, low-fat dairy products, fish, eggs, soy, and only occasionally meat.

A diet thus conceived, definitely avoids specific nutrients whose role in the pathogenesis of cardiovascular diseases is suggested by several experimental studies. Among the latter, those that have investigated the metabolic effects of the intake of sugars such as **sucrose** (compound formed from one molecule of glucose and one of fructose) and **fructose**, show a significant correlation with weight gain, also suggesting a possible role in the increase of triglycerides and blood pressure.

Other studies show that excess of salt and partially hydrogenated fatty acids found in margarine and many pastry products, promote the **atherosclerotic process** and favor the **meta-**

bolic syndrome.

In 1998 the World Health Organization (WHO) proposed a first **definition of the metabolic syndrome** which was followed by others, which differ in the type and number of variables considered and in the levels of cut-off (threshold values) used.

The best known definition, applied in clinical practice is that of the National Cholesterol Education Program Adult Treatment Panel (ATP) III of 2001. It does not consider any direct or indirect diagnostic element of insulin resistance, but contemplates the presence of three variables simultaneously present between the following: **abdominal obesity, high blood pressure, hypertriglyceridemia, low HDL cholesterol and blood glucose> 110 mg / dl (also including diabetes).**

In **2005**, the International Diabetes Federation (IDF) stepped in with its own definition.

It is characterized by placing the **visceral obesity** as an essential element to which you must add two other criteria among the customary ones (hypertriglyceridemia, low HDL cholesterol, hypertension, hyperglycemia, including diabetes).

About 1 month after the publication of the IDF criteria, the American Heart Association and the National Heart, Lung and Blood Institute issued a statement on the metabolic syndrome, which has expanded the ATP III criteria, bringing the level diagnostic blood glucose from 110 to **100 mg/dl**[62][63].

In persons with metabolic syndrome, **the risk of cardiovascular mortality doubles** and there is a **fivefold increase in the risk of developing diabetes.**

In contrast, the consumption of **omega-3 fatty acids**, which are rich particularly in blue fish (rich in DHA and EPA) and in wild herbs (rich in a-linolenic acid), as well as in specific phyto-

---

62 http://www.giornaledicardiologia.it/r.php?v=661&a=7716&l=10695&f=allegati/00661_2010_11/fulltext/S1-11_2010_08_29-32.pdf, last access 15.10.2015.
63 La sindrome metabolica: impatto sul rischio cardiovascolare, Fiocca et al., G Ital Cardiol 2010; 11 (11 Suppl 1): 29S-32S

chemicals compounds present in plants, holds an anti-inflammatory and antithrombotic function.

The previously described food pattern aligns with the results of several epidemiological studies which have clearly shown that individuals who adopt a **predominantly vegetarian diet** with unprocessed whole foods, have a lower risk of developing cardiovascular disease, compared with people who adopt a Western diet, rich in flour and refined grains, animal protein, saturated fat, trans fats and salt.

It is increasingly evident the above mentioned diet evokes the **traditional Mediterranean diet**, prior to the revolution of the food industry; a diet based mainly on plant foods, which provides a daily intake of low-glycemic grains (whole wheat bread and pasta made from durum wheat semolina), vegetables, even wild, fresh fruit and nuts (walnuts, almonds, hazelnuts, pistachios, pine nuts, flax seeds, sesame, sunflower and pumpkin), extra virgin olive oil, and as a protein source mainly legumes, fish, some dairy, modest consumption of wine and only occasionally, meat.

The traditional Mediterranean diet taken as a whole including its potential conviviality, biodiversity, seasonality, was recognized by the United Nations Educational, Scientific and Cultural Organization (UNESCO), **as cultural heritage for humanity.**

This diet has been proven effective in **reducing body weight, blood glucose and insulin resistance, dyslipidemia, hypertension, type 2 diabete**s, metabolic syndrome and inflammation. In fact, clinical trials conducted on subjects at high cardiovascular risk investigating the effects of the Mediterranean diet, showed a reduced incidence of cardiovascular disease. A clinical study in patients suffering from myocardial infarction has moreover established the possible secondary preventive role of the Mediterranean diet. Ultimately, adhering to a Mediterranean diet first of all translates into predominantly feeding of foods of plant origin and, therefore, not only in increasing the proportion of fiber, but also antioxidants, anti-inflammatory and immunomodulatory activities. The Mediterranean diet does not provide for a certain reduction of intake of total fat, the percentage of which can provide 25-35% of total dietary calories, but provides for a **reduction of saturated fatty acids** (which are rich in **meats, cold cuts and dairy** products in particular).

Parallelly, the Mediterranean diet allows to **increase** the consumption of foods high in **monounsaturated and polyunsaturated fatty acids**. Monounsaturated Fatty Acids (indicated with the acronym MUFA) are fatty acids characterized by having only one double bond among all present between the various carbon atoms; differ in this from the saturated fatty acids (which possess only single bonds) and polyunsaturated (which instead have numerous double bonds)[64].

Polyunsaturated fatty acids can assume **cis or trans** conformation depending on the conformal geometry of the molecule.

Important series of fats belong to this family, such as **omega-3**, omega-6 and omega-9.

The increase in monounsaturated and polyunsaturated fatty acids results in a lowering of the **LDL cholesterol** blood concentration, and emerges as an effective strategy for the reduction of cardiovascular risks.

In the food sector, **monounsaturated fatty acids** are found mainly in olive oil and peanut oil and in lower percentages also in all other vegetable oils of various seeds.

Polyunsaturated fatty acids are found in good quantity in fish oil, in seed oils with different percentages for the omega-3 (prevailing in linseed and sesame seeds oils) and omega-6 (prevalent in sunflower, corn and soya oil, in which, however, there is also a good percentage of n-3), in the oil seeds and in certain wild herbs.

Already considered the elixir of youth and health since the times of ancient Greece, **olive oil,** according to recent epidemiological solid results, in clinical trials (PREDIMED) and cohort

---

64 https://it.wikipedia.org/wiki/Acidi_grassi_monoinsaturi , last access 17.10. 2015

study (EPIC), confirms to be preventive against various factors risk of cardiovascular disease, such as diabetes, obesity and metabolic syndrome. In addition, it is a confirmed promoter of an increase in the longevity, not only in function of the ascertained cardioprotective role, which is expressed in an improvement of the lipid profile, of the endothelial function, of inflammation and thrombosis; but also showing an effect of secondary prevention in cases of myocardial strokes. These potential benefits can be explained in several experimental studies, which demonstrate that specific components of olive oil have antihypertensive effect, antithrombotic, antioxidant, anti-inflammatory and, as recent data suggest, anticarcinogenic. Traditionally, the beneficial effects of olive oil are attributed to high content of monounsaturated fatty acids, of which the main one, with a percentage ranging between 55-83% of the total fatty acid content, is oleic acid. It is a fatty acid capable of influencing the expression of certain genes, where the increase of plasma concentration is associated with a reduction in the incidence of metabolic syndrome. Indeed, monounsaturated fatty acids improve glucose metabolism, increase postprandial fat oxidation and thermogenesis induced by diet, being able therefore to counter the increase of body weight. But in addition to oleic acid, olive oil, contains a mixture of many other bioactive chemical compounds (tocopherols, squalene, sterols, terpenes, pigments), including also hydrophilic compounds called polyphenols, important at preventive level thanks to their potentiality of reducing inflammation, platelet aggregation, the oxidative stress of the cell (and therefore any of ROS damage to DNA), as well as serving a proapoptotic function. Of course the phenolic compounds are present predominantly in virgin and extra virgin olive oils, obtained by a mechanical pressing of the olives and cold extracts, while refining processes will certainly cut down the content.

As for the **dried fruit consumption**, several epidemiological studies have shown that regular consumption lowers cardiovascular risk (in the context of PREDIMED study it is highlighted in participants assigned to the intervention group of the Mediterranean diet supplemented with nuts, a decrease in cardiovascular mortality by 55% , and a reduction of the prevalence of the metabolic syndrome or regression of such illness), but also of total mortality.

Clinical trials have shown that consumption of nuts protects against cardiovascular risk through **several mechanisms**: by regulating inflammatory processes, oxidative stress, endothelial functions and enhancing the multiple cardiovascular risk factors, namely significantly reducing LDL cholesterol and lowering blood pressure. The dried fruit is a "dense" food from the energy point of view, as it is rich in fat. However, it's inclusion in a proper dietary pattern does not show a significant increase in weight. Conversely an inverse relationship between consumption of nuts, BMI and abdominal adiposity has been observed. This presumably is due to greater thermogenic effect induced by high content of monounsaturated and polyunsaturated fats, for reduced accessibility to intestinal enzymes of fat content in nuts, for a greater satiating effect than any other equivalent snack, rich in carbohydrates and/or saturated fat. Dried fruits are rich in monounsaturated and polyunsaturated fatty acids (in particular among the latter the α-linolenic acid most abundant in nuts, precursor of n-3 fatty acids called EPA and DHA) of insoluble fiber, protein, minerals such as magnesium and potassium, phytosterols, tocopherols and polyphenols.

In the context of a meal rich in carbohydrates, the simultaneous intake of nuts reduces peak postprandial glucose, therefore also potentially representing benefits to **diabetics**.

As opposed to nutrients that have a protective function, there are specific nutrients that instead have a **role in the pathogenesis** of chronic degenerative diseases, especially cardiovascular diseases.

In relation to this, recent studies report a 24% increase in cardiovascular risk for each increment of 2% of the intake of **trans fatty acids** (abundant in **margarines** but also present in some ready meals, sauces and **pastries**, and though scarcely in meat ruminant animals, milk and dairy products. This figure can be explained by the high degree of atherogenicity, even for low consumption. Trans fatty acids promote dyslipidemia, increasing the levels of LDL cholesterol and decreasing those of HDL cholesterol. Certainly, the percentage of macronutrients is important in prevention.

With this regard, the European EPIC study has showed that an **excess of protein** (18-20%) is associated with weight gain and obesity.

Recent studies have also revealed the importance of the distribution of calories during the day, or the frequency of the meals, as well as the potential of fasting, all factors that may substantially have a beneficial effect. **Fasting for 24 hours** intermittently, in animal models, reduces inflammation and oxidative stress, protecting against obesity, diabetes and hypertension. A clinical study in obese or overweight premenopausal women, showed, following a two-day non-consecutive fasting in a week, a reduction in body weight, fat mass, waist circumference, LDL cholesterol, triglycerides, and PCR blood pressure and clinical trials being conducted in non-obese showed improvement in cardiovascular risk factors.

Cancer prevention through diet

On October 14st, 2014 the 'International Agency for Research on Cancer (IARC), published the latest revision of the European Code Against Cancer (ECAC), a series of recommendations to be adopted in order to significantly reduce the risk of cancer. The team involved more than 150 researchers, epidemiologists and biologists, responsible for collecting and reviewing scientific data judged convincing. These data, also obtained by imposing prospective studies, both European and American, have investigated the relationship between diet and cancer, enlisting hundreds of thousands of healthy volunteers. The participants all underwent a blood sampling and nutrition questionnaires, con-

firming that by adhering to the ECAC nutritional recommenda-
tions, **it is feasible to prevent one third of malign cancers,** thus
reducing cancer mortality, **as well as for cardiovascular diseases.**
Nutritional recommendations of ECAC state[65]:
- Eat plenty of whole grains, legumes, vegetables and fruits
- Mitigate high calorie density foods (high in sugar and fat)
- Limit red meat
- Avoid preserved meat
- Avoid sugary drinks
- limit salt-rich foods.

At first glance, it is first of all clear that a diet based on
ECAC recommendations, does not presumably contain a large
percentage of **saturated fatty acids**.

It presupposes, in fact, a limited consumption of **red meat**
(a quantity not exceeding 300 g. per week was significantly protective for colorectal cancer) and the more of preserved meat (of
which laboration involves the addition of nitrites/nitrates, from
which carcinogenic nitrosamines can generate; the smoking, or
the adding of salt, which can contribute to the development of
stomach cancer) for which the data show an increase in stomach
and colorectal cancer risk. The WHO in 2002 had suggested to
limit the consumption of red meat.

Examples of **preserved meats** are hot dogs, canned or
salted meat, as well as ready-made or sauces in which meat is
processed The WHO, through the IARC (International Agency for
Research on Cancer) has formalized the scientific evidence
emerged under the association between the consumption of red
meat, processed meats and carcinogenesis. The IARC fact, whose
job is also to classify according to the scientific strength of evidence the various potential carcinogens agents[66], has included in
Group 1 preserved meat, as **carcinogen** for humans.

This means that solid scientific evidence has clearly

65 www.dietandcancerreport.org, last access 17.10.015
66 http://monographs.iarc.fr/ENG/Classification/index.php,ast access
17.10.015

demonstrated the ability of this food to increase the risk of **colorectal cancer** in individuals exposed to a specific use and for a specific time, a risk that increases with its consumption.

Specifically, an analysis of the data of 10 studies estimates that the **daily consumption of a portion of 50 gr. of processed meats** increases the risk of colorectal cancer by **18%**.

As for red meat, the classification in the 2A group is derived from the observation of an association between consumption and cancer of the colon and rectum (also with some relationship with pancreatic cancer and prostate), but with still limited scientific evidence. The classification of the final IARC, validating the recommendation to **limit consumption of red meat and only occasionally consume preserved meat** (especially since even in economically weaker countries the habit of increasingly consuming meat) provides an opportunity to identify possible guidelines related to the consumption of these foods, that are able to maximize the benefits and minimize the risks. This remains inextricably linked to the need for appropriate treatment for these foods (cooking the meat at high temperatures causes e.g. the formation of carcinogenic polycyclic aromatic hydrocarbons) and the adoption of a dietary pattern that still allows for taking antioxidants capable of protecting the risk, as shown by ECAC.

The diet recommended by ECAC allows a modest amount of **sugars**, (the WHO recommends that the sugar taken daily is not more than 5% of the total calorie consumption) with particular emphasis on the limitation apart from of high-calorie foods, the consumption of sugary drinks (fruit juices, soft drinks, snacks, yogurt liquids, alcohol) that are among the foods that primarily cause obesity. Recent studies have in fact shown that sugary drinks induce less satiety compared to an isoenergetic amount of carbohydrates in the solid state. In addition, the fructose often present in these drinks, (as well as in syrups commonly used in the food industry) increases insulin resistance, increases liver fat synthesis, inducing an increase in blood levels of triglycerides and uric acid. The latter, besides increasing prevalence of gout, is capable of mediating vasoconstriction and therefore the increase in blood pressure.

The recommended dietary pattern, is certainly rich in **plant foods**, thanks to the daily intake of whole grains, legumes, fruits and vegetables. A food pattern thus conceived, that respects the typical varieties of each season[67] and preserve as much as possible the contents in phytochemical compounds, of which plants, if cultivated in a natural way without synthetic pesticides, are particularly rich in. In addition to supporting the maintenance of a favourable body weight, it especially helps, through treatment and adequate cooking, to put in the dish a real anti-cancer cocktail. This is effective through daily intake of vitamins, minerals and antioxidants thanks to the contribution of polyphenols.

Among the phytochemicals, **polyphenols** have detoxifying antiproliferative, anti inflammatory, anti-angiogenic functions and are capable of acting for protective purposes, to the gene expression level. Polyphenols act specifically, being able to interfere each in different stages of carcinogenesis. Consequently, only an intake of various foods containing them and perhaps an integration of different cuisines, both Oriental and European, can promote increased tumor countering power, thanks to the 'action of these substances.

Specifically, adhering to the first recommendation certainly allows a good supply of fibers that first of all increase intestinal motility, accelerating the transit and therefore decreasing the contact time of any carcinogenic substances with the mucosa. Moreover, the **plant fibers**, as a result of bacterial fermentation, originate the short-chain fatty acid capable to block cell proliferation. Studies show in particular that vegetable consumption is inversely associated with the risk of lung cancer, in which,

---

67

http://www.istitutotumori.mi.it/upload_files/Spunti_per_una_varieta_di_cereali_e_legumi_D5.pd for the same consumer, it is the variability of vegetables to support greater protection. Such prevention is also confirmed for defence from bowel cancer (for which the fiber from cereals results extremely protective) and from breast cancer. Prospective studies confirm a consumption of fruit provides protection from cancer of the esophagus, stomach and upper respiratory tract. The recommendation provides a daily intake of at least 600g. of fruit and vegetables, which, associated with whole grains and legumes (low glycemic index foods), helps to reduce the size and speed of the intestinal absorption of glucose, which results in a reduction in postprandial glycaemia.

This is an important finding because several studies now show a link between higher values of glucose (albeit in the normal range) and increased risk of developing various cancers (including breast cancer, colorectal and pancreas) as well as a prognostic role in blood sugar and insulin, particularly for cancers of the breast and colon. A lower blood glucose in normal levels, can help to starve the cancer cells, glucose-hungry, but especially helps to keep down the secretion of **insulin**, a hormone that can influence directly and indirectly on carcinogenesis. Insulin, in fact, by promoting the increase of growth hormone receptors, stimulates the synthesis of insulin-like growth factors (IGF-I), essential for tumor development, the promoters of cell cycle progression, angiogenesis and metastatic activity.

Furthermore, insulin regulates the production of vascular growth factors and hormones of the adipose tissue. Therefore, in the context of cancer prevention, it may be useful to **inhibit the increase of IGF-I**, increasing the consumption of low-glycemic index foods, containing high-index foods blood insulin and moderating the protein contribution (amino acid specific), which is correlated directly with the synthesis of IGF-I.

In conclusion, taking into account what is indicated by the results of the most convincing studies that investigated the relationship between diet and risk of chronic degenerative diseases, adopting an **appropriate nutrition habit**, emerges among the basic prerequisites for the achievement of the wonderful hope of the disease "zero" through nutritional prevention, enabled by the introduction of protective foods and avoiding or limiting the intake of foods that promote the development of diseases[68].

---

68 www.sanostiledivita.it//drive/File/strategy_english_OMS.pdf, last access 1.11.2015

5.7 Cardiovascular and oncological risks

Francesca Mirabelli

Cardiovascular and oncological diseases in Italy represent, respectively, the **first and the second leading cause of death and disability**.

The World Health Organization states that "**ischemic heart disease** is currently the leading cause of death in the world; It is increasing and has become a real epidemic that knows no borders. "

Cardiovascular diseases affect both the masculine and the feminine; it was estimated that among the **European population under 75**, cardiovascular diseases are responsible for 42% of deaths among males and 38% among females.

Both cardiovascular disease and the cancer diseases are known to be associated with **risk factors** on which it is theoretically possible to act in order to reduce the incidence of the disease itself: they are closely related to **lifestyle**, **tobacco** use, to **incorrect food habits, physical inactivity**, psychosocial **stress**.

The World Health Organization has stated that more than **three quarters** of global cardiovascular deaths can be prevented by implementing **lifestyle** modifications.

Cardiovascular prevention is therefore a major challenge for the general population, for health professionals and for the public health administrators and consists of a series of coordinated actions at the individual, social and public levels aimed at minimizing the impact of cardiovascular diseases and related disabilities.

Preventive actions should be continued throughout life, **from birth** (if not sooner!) until old age. As stated by the European guidelines for prevention of cardiovascular diseases[69] and

---

69 European Guidelines on CVD Prevention in Clinical Practice. Eur H Journal 2012

as reaffirmed in the 'European Charter for Health of the Heart "[70], which was ratified in the European Parliament in June 2007.

The elements needed to achieve cardiovascular health are as follows:

- Not **smoking**
- Avoiding **alcohol** abuse
- Avoiding a **sedentary** lifestyle, being physically active, practicing an appropriate sport: at least 30 minutes of moderate aerobic activity five times a week (brisk walking, running, swimming, cycling. .)
- Following a correct **nutrition**, low in salt and animal fats, rich in fruits and vegetables
- Avoiding being **overweight**
- Keeping **blood pressure** below 140/90 mmHg
- Keeping total **cholesterol levels** to below 190 mg / dL (for the general population)
- Maintaining a normal **glucose metabolism**
- Avoiding excessive **stress**.

Theoretically, prevention begins during pregnancy and continues until death. In daily practice preventive interventions are usually directed to men and women of middle or old age, and are limited among the young or very old. A healthy lifestyle in the first decades of life is fundamental: an increasing number of evidence has shown that **cardiovascular risk** begins to increase at an early, if not young, age. Even the lack of attention to the prevention of cardiovascular disease in the elderly has proved unjustified. Several studies have shown that preventive measures (such as lowering of blood pressure and smoking cessation) are useful up to advanced ages.

The reduction of cardiovascular risk is a winning strategy in terms of public health and resource optimization: it can lead to cost savings arising from the number of **cardiovascular events**

---

70 European Heart Network. European Cardiovascular Disease Statistics. 2008 edition

avoided, by the reduction of drug costs and health benefits necessary for the treatment and follow -up of the affected individual; can result in cost savings arising from a minor loss of productivity in individuals of working age affected by the disease; It can exert a preventive action to other conditions that have **similar etiology** such as **cancer**, **lung disease**, **diabetes type 2**; It can improve the quality and duration of life of people[71].

---

71 National Institute for Health and Clinical Excellence. Prevention of Cardiovascular Disease: Costing Report. 2010. Nice Public Health Guidance 25

5.8 Psychiatric Risk
Angela Meggiolaro

We **distinguish**:
-   Concomitant factors: sex age, class, immigration and urbanization
-   Predisposing factors: prenatal and perinatal complications, viral infections, genetics
-   Precipitating Factors: stressful life events, conditions related to development, use of drugs.

In the monitoring of **work-related stress**, the way work is designed, organized and managed, is related to risks that may increase the level of stress and can cause major effects on mental and physical health of workers[72]. It can, in fact, prevent and manage psychosocial risks related to job stress.

The European Union, in fact, pays attention to this issue by including it among the objectives to be achieved through the **Europe 2020** Strategy, in order to ensure the health and welfare of workers throughout their working lives.

On the topic, Eurofound (European Foundation for the Improvement of Living and Working Conditions) published a report entitled "Psychosocial risks in Europe -Prevalence and strategies for prevention" by combining data of Eurofound itself and EU-OSHA (**European Agency for Safety and Health at Work**). The presented data analysis the exposure to psychosocial risks on the part of workers, and how this is associated to their health, including information on the commitment of managers in preventing psychosocial risks in their companies and what are the types of companies in which they implement measures to prevent these

---

72 cfr. M. Giovannone, I rischi psicosociali: un focus sullo stress lavoro – correlato, Literature Review, Literature Review, in Bollettino ADAPT, n. 15/2010

risks[73].

Among psychiatric disorders, **schizophrenia** presents risk factors based on scientific evidence.

---

73 http://www.bollettinoadapt.it/la-prevenzione-dei-rischi-psicosociali-europa/ , last access 02.09.2015

5.9 Genetic Risk
Angela Meggiolaro

After the completion of the **mapping** of the human **genome** in the context of the Human Genome Project in **2001**, the genome analysis has acquired a specific role relevant to the advancement of medicine and health care: genomics and molecular genetics have developed rapidly[74]. Consequently, the last decade has witnessed a growing and uncontrolled availability of genetic testing for diseases not only monogenic, but also complex[75].

The Centers for Disease Control (CDC) indicate genomic alterations as a contributory cause in nine of the ten leading causes of death in the United States, with particular reference to **cancer** and **cardiovascular disease**. These diseases arise from the interaction between genetic risk factors, environmental and behavioral elements, including nutrition and physical activity. In addition, a large proportion of pediatric hospitalizations are due to diseases affected by genetic susceptibility (eg. Birth defects, allergic diseases). It is estimated that the risk of developing a certain disease at least in part genetically is about 5% before the age of 25 and increases to 65% or more over a lifetime. So, although the dominant role of environmental risk factors over genetic ones has been reaffirmed, it is now established that the risk of disease stems from the mutual interaction the different causes.

There is increasingly demand in the US for **online genetic testing**, available directly to consumers without a prescription,

---

74 La Genomica in Sanità Pubblica sintesi delle evidenze e delle conoscenze disponibili sull'utilizzo della genomica ai fini della prevenzione. IJPH - 2012, Volume 9, Number 1, Suppl. 1
75 Van El CG, Cornel MC, Genetic testing and common disorders in a public health framework. Recommendations of the European Society of Human Genetics. European Journal of Human Genetics 2011; 19: 377–381

without passing a careful evaluation of the clinical validity and utility by experienced professionals. The simple analytical validity of a test (assuming it has been evaluated with due care) is not sufficient to establish the real utility. Therefore, premature commercialization of these tests should also be carefully considered in light of the possible negative consequences.

After studying monogenic and chromosomal disorders in the second half of the twentieth century, in the last two decades of research in genetics and genomics, the focus has increasingly turned to common complex diseases. For complex disease is intended all diseases caused by variables, including a **multifactorial etiology** as monogenic subset. When speaking of "susceptibility genes", we refer to genetic variants with low predictive value[76].

Currently, genetic tests in use principally ragard rare hereditary diseases, mostly Mendelian, although there are some significant exceptions related to multifactorial diseases. Unlike what occurs for a high predictive genes value, such as susceptibility to breast cancer (**BRCA1** and **BRCA2**) or colorectal cancer, the transfer in clinical practice of the discoveries relating to tests that analyze low gene variants predictive value is problematic.

The main criterion for evaluating the real benefits of applying a genetic test (for a gene or group of genes) of susceptibility to complex diseases is its **predictive ability** at the population level. Moreover, an intervention, to be effective, must be available on a large scale. It is important to emphasize that the polymorphisms that confer susceptibility are distributed differently in populations, so their predictive value is measured in the different ethnic groups before you can use this information for diagnostic purposes.

In recent years, studies regarding the relationship between lifestyles, environmental factors and individual genotype

---

76 Recommendations of the European Society of Human Genetics Carla G van El and Martina C Cornel on behalf of the ESHG Public and Professional Policy Committee

led to the development of a series of **genetic tests** whose reliability and usefulness have yet to be evaluated and validated. The Human Genetics Commission in 2009 added the following types of tests:

• Test on behaviors and lifestyles, aimed at obtaining information about the behavioral inclinations, abilities (physical or cognitive), the response to certain environmental conditions of a person, to assist in modifying performance through deliberate behavioral changes;

• Nutrigenetic tests, aimed at getting the individual metabolism information with regarding to food assumption;

• Phenotypic tests, aimed at obtaining information on the phenotype of an individual is influenced by genotype (eg. Tests indicating the genetic basis of a person's eye color).

The existence of the genetic component in diseases was suggested as a result of an observed recurrence of cases of disease in families than the general population and the correlation to the character between genetically identical twins than non-identical twins or siblings.

The determination of a character is the result of a myriad of genes, each with different and specific function. The identification of the individual functional contribution to the development of the disease is intuitively investigable[77].

The identification of genes involved in complex disease for mutations may offer the possibility of prevention through the determination of individual genetic risk factors.

---

77 PIGNATTI, P. F. Malattie genetiche multifattoriali. Riv Med Lab - JLM, Vol. 4, S.1, 2003

Table I: example of mutations in complex diseases. Taken from:
Botstein & Risch, Nature Genetics Suppl 2003; 33:228.

DISEASE	GENE/MUTATION	RR
Alzheimer	APOE e4	4-15
Trombosis	V Leiden Factor	5-10
NIDDM	PPARγ P12A	1,25
IDDM	INS VNTR prom	1,5-2,5
Crohn	NOD2 G908R	6
Ca Breast	BRCA2 N372H	1,3
Ca colon	APC I130K	2
	MTHFR C677T	2

The reported **relative risks** are low, and vary from 1.25 to 10 in various cases. The data of genetic risk relative to developing a multifactorial disease, can form the basis for the development of a genetic susceptibility testing.

The frequency of the diseases under **predictive genetic tests** in the most economically developed societies and the great individual variability in response to drugs now put these tests in the interest of research and development, as is also evident from the last Italian census of genetic tests carried out to by the Italian society of Human Genetics[78]. Among the genetic tests, the most carried out in Italy in 2000, were HLA and cystic fibrosis.

The individual genotyping to determine the **hereditary predisposition** to complex **diseases** or altered responses to drugs must be entrusted to the free individual decision after receiving appropriate information, supported by the necessary interpretative competence and relational specialist, respecting the confidentiality of information.

In the new field of genomic medicine, the deepening of the knowledge of the **links between genetic abnormalities and environmental triggers** is convincing scientists that although the

---

78 http://sigu.univr.it consultato , last access 02.09. 2015

disease can be classified into broad categories, in every individual a disease presents unique traits, although losing diagnose as the expression of a defined disease in general terms. Genetic medicine is exploring a new customized approach to the disease, in which the problem of each patient is treated as an "orphan" disease.

Thanks to **the drop in DNA sequencing costs**, we see the formation of an archive of big data that people can use to contact people with a similar **genetic profile** to theirs. In the future, when these archives will be expanded and it will become possible to test the entire sequence of human DNA, millions of people will be able to search within healthcare networks directed by the patient, subjects that have genetic elements in common between them, discussing about their diseases and collaborating in the search for therapeutic solutions.

These commons oriented health patients will also be able to generate a lateral growth enough to bring to public attention the disease they are dealing. This enhances their potential to **intensify the pressure on governments**, the academic community and private companies to potentiate research on various diseases, as well as to finance research, clinical studies and therapeutic solutions.

Individuals with **biological affinity** who joined on the basis of DNA can also use big data to cross the data about each other's lifestyles - eating habits, smoking and drinks, exercise, working environment. This could, consequently allow identifying correlations between certain genetic predispositions and different environmental triggers as these aggregations of related human types contemplate also a history of the various existences - from prenatal life to old age, even to death - will become quite possible to develop algorithms capable of signaling the potential risk of disease in different stages of life and to suggest effective therapies.

It is estimated that around the middle of this century, if not before, each person will have the opportunity to access the search engine of a global health commons, to register their **genetic configuration**, locate a group of people with similar genomes to, to receive a detailed report on the disturbances that could threaten one's health over the life course and to have personalized information on the most effective medical treatment to heal and stay healthy; all this at almost zero marginal cost.

5.10 Dentistry risk and zero cavity
Eloisa Fioravanti

The concept of "**health**", based on the definition of the WHO entails "a state of complete physical, mental and social wellness, not just the absence of disease", for over 50 years it therefore covers all specialties of medical science and helps to develop new research and studies of therapy and prevention of diseases.

Since 1984 also an enhancement of health promotion process has begun, that "gives people the ability to increase and improve control over their health": the individual thereby becomes active and integral part of a broader process, shared and communitary, which horizontally includes the physician, the patient, the community and the state system, in a virtuous circle based on sharing responsibilities, with a view towards the reduction of disease.

In 2007, the General Assembly of the WHO added **oral health** among the main elements for the achievement of the global health and defined the priority areas of action for its improvement: effective use of **fluoride**, power control and nutrition, control of **oral hygiene** habits and **tobacco** use, oral health monitoring in children and prevention of oral diseases. The development of dental science is a great example of a how careful prevention campaign has managed to decrease in thirty years the cavity disease with consequent benefit in terms of global health and economic savings.

Towards the beginning of the sixties, epidemiological studies singled out **caries** as the most common chronic disease in the world, covering over **90% of adults**, with considerable repercussions on the health and welfare of the individual. In 1978 the WHO raised awareness among national health systems by engaging in policies of prevention and protection of oral health: Goal were set for 2000 and 2020, aimed at checking and clearing of the risk of tooth decay.

Year 2000	Year 2020
50% of children of 5-6 years without cavities	95% of children of 5-6 years without cavity
DMFT <3 to 12 years of age	DMFT <0,7 to 12 years of age
85% of the population of 18 years of age with all the elements present	95% of the population of 18 years of age with all the elements present
75% of the population of 35-45 years with at least 20 elements	75% of the population of 35-45 years with at least 20 elements
50% of the population over 65 years with at least 20 elements	50% of the population over 65 years with at least 20 elements

(Table retrieved from Polimeni, Pediatric Dentistry, Elsevier 2012)

As shown in the reported table, the objectives are very ambitious, affecting the pediatric and adult population. taking into consideration the DMFT index, the index of occurrence of cavity (acronym for **Decayed, Missing, Filled Teeth**, ie the sum of decayed teeth, missing or blocked on the number of subjects).

Tooth decay is in fact the trigger for the onset of an oral disease that also involves other elements (tooth loss and the need for dental treatment, even in acute) with significant consequences on the economic and health costs.

By **definition, caries** is multifactorial chronic degenerative and transmissible disease which covers the hard tissues of the tooth. It is still one of the most prevalent pathologies both in the pediatric population as in the adult, despite the preventive and information campaigns, who can not, however, act simultaneously on all the aetiological variables.

Four variables are triggers and **causes**, tightly interconnected together:
· **bacterial plaque** (microbiological component)
· **Diet** (eating habits)
· host susceptibility (**genetic** predisposition and variable)
· **Time**

The disease is in fact established when there is an imbalance between the host flora of the oral cavity and the cariogenic bacterial strains, which increase and generate the initial injury, represented by a continuous solution of the hard tooth tissue. This **imbalance** is favored when, over time, a complex interaction is established between the cariogenic bacteria, fermentable carbohydrates introduced the subject and host factors, such as saliva or other diseases. Many studies have also highlighted the close correlation between the onset of the disease and the socio-economic and cultural level of the individual, and its uncontrolled spread especially in urban and industrialized areas.

It can be talked about a real beginning of the disease since the Industrial Revolution and the introduction of refined sugar in the diet, as early as 1700. It is curious to verify that in fact, according to ethno-paleontological studies, tooth decay is a **"recent" disease**, inextricably linked to the Western industrialization process. Few traces of cavity go back to the Greek-Roman or medieval times (related to the use of other sweeteners), as it begins to appear in the upper class with the introduction of sugar, while it is absent for a long time in the eastern populations (who routinely use tea, food rich in fluorine, a carious protective element) or in those in Africa.

Obviously, it is utopian to think you can control all the etiological factors simultaneously and, although **the idea of a vaccine** against the microorganisms responsible for the lesion **is still far** from reality (difficult due to the variety of strains and the differences in harmful actions on teeth). Research, however, has been addressed to act on the control of eating habits and prevention at different levels.

The most extensive and widespread preventive measure concerns the **fluoridation** of domestic water, which has led to a reduction of the diseases, despite the increase of production and consumption of cariogenic foods. Prevention guidelines of oral health in Italian and American pediatrics (free to download and available at the following addresses: http://www.aapd.org/policies/ and http://www.sioi.it/?page_id=1795), constantly updated and reviewed with scientific evidence of the moment, are in fact recommending to national governments to introduce fluoride in drinking water in order to strengthen the tooth structure and make it less susceptible to acid demineralization by the cariogenic bacteria. In addition, it is recommended to take fluoride, systemic and topical, both in children and in pregnant women and to carry out the sealing of the first permanent molars already at school age. However the controlled intake of fluoride can not be enough to prevent the risk of disease, therefore it but must still be associated with the instruction of home oral hygiene practices and proper nutrition.

Daily use of fluoride toothpaste and toothbrushes to remove food debris, periodic visits to the dentist and information campaigns can help raise the focus on achieving the goals proposed by the WHO. Furthermore, a varied **diet** low in complex carbohydrates, particularly avoiding gummy or sticky foods (which maintain on the tooth surface the harmful substances, inhibiting the physiological self-adhering which occurs during chewing), helping to prevent the onset of cavities and other systemic diseases.

The multifactorial nature of the carious disease makes it an excellent model for an example of "zero" system: the base is placed on **prevention**, which must become more and more informed shared alliance between doctor, patient and health care system.

Tooth decay in childhood as in adulthood, triggers a mechanism of absence of global health that can have **different outcomes**: the disease is painful and can have acute occurings that require emergency treatment (pulpits), or chronic phenomena leading to the necrosis of the vital pulp of the tooth and the loss of the elements, resulting in physical and emotional harms. Dental care, long and expensive, does not reduce the risk of the disease, which can develop again if the approach mode isn't altered. Therapy, in fact, does not represent the proper way to eliminate tooth decay, while a proper primary prevention, secondary and tertiary education could nullify the risk of onset.

Therefore, In a **"zero action"** optic, the state system is committed to ensuring the fluoridation of drinking water and information, including through awareness-raising campaigns, specialist visits in schools and widespread dissemination of recommendations (also via new media, useful also in this case for their ability to connect skills and experience); clinical strengthening of the patient's motivation and making periodic visits screening and possibly allowing early detection of disease. While the patient is given the task of taking care of oral hygiene and personal diet.

In this perspective, the spending (biological and economic) is reduced to a minimum both for the individual and for the state, triggering a virtuous cycle with as main and co-responsible actors, the patient and the doctor, both are united in a tendency to decrease the risk and reset pathology.

6. The paradigm of communication and doctor Google
Bruno Corda, Angelo Barbato, Angela Meggiolaro

With the development of the third industrial revolution, starting in about 1970, information technology has produced a worldwide network of public access computers: **Internet!**

Since then, communication has become increasingly multi-channelled and more and more real time. On September 15th, 1997 **Google** was launched, later becoming the search engine that changed the world.

As well as cataloguing and indexing the resources of the World Wide Web, **Google** has started to work on maps (Google Maps), email (Gmail), photos, online sales, translations, videos and programs specifically created.

It is the most visited site in the world[79], so popular that different languages have developed new denomination **verbs** from his mark, with the meaning of search with Google or, more generally, to search the web. Among the neologisms we find for example the verb, "to google", also translatable, for instance, in Italian "googlare"[80] and German "googeln"[81].

Google, as expected due to its universal character even in the medical field, began to be **Dr. Google.**

The first big break in this field has been to open to different views and interpretations spaces.

This gives the opportunity to everyone, both patient and health care worker, to confront a variety of information. It has been made possible to **expand the knowledge** up to a level of detail such as to representing a use not only to laymen but also for the professionals.

---

79 http://www.alexa.com/siteinfo/google.com, last access 27.10. 2015

80 http://www.treccani.it/vocabolario/googlare_%28Neologismi%29/ , last access 27.10. 2015

81 https://it.wikipedia.org/wiki/Google consultato 27 agosto 2015

Since August 2015 Google is no longer enough, Larry Page and Sergey Brin, founders of the Mountain View giant Google launched a home-revolution, a radical restructuring, overcoming of the model Google and the birth of the **Alphabet** galaxy. This creates a new corporate structure that separates the research on the web, YouTube with research and investment. Alphabet, the new holding company, contains a "collection" of companies, the largest of which is Google itself.

As for the medical field, particularly in research against aging and in the study of age-related diseases such as Alzheimer, Google has already created the company Ca.Li.Co. (**California Life Company**).

Ca.Li.Co. is a research and development company whose aim is to take advantage of advanced technologies to increase the understanding of the biological mechanisms that control the lifespan. The knowledge gained will be used to develop interventions that enable people to lead a healthier and longer life. This mission will require an unprecedented level of interdisciplinary effort with a long-term orientation, for which funding is already in place[82].

Ca.Li.Co. is the life sciences company supported by Google, led by CEO (Chief Executive Officer) Arthur D. Levinson, Ph.D. (Former President and CEO of Genentech) and Hal V. Barron, MD (former Executive Vice President and Chief Medical Officer of Genentech). The agreement paves the way for Ca.Li.Co. to establish a center for worldwide research and development in the Bay Area of San Francisco[83].

As already stated there is an ongoing new market transition where traditional multinational capitalist (**Abbvie**) start to work with emerging companies in the sharing economy and commons (Ca.Li.Co.).

This is the case of **Abbvie**, a global biopharmaceutical company, research-based and established in 2013 after the sepa-

82 http://www.calicolabs.com/ , last access 27.08.2015
83 http://www.calicolabs.com/news/2014/09/03/ last access 27.08.2015

ration from Abbott Laboratories. The company's mission is to develop and commercialize therapies that address complex diseases. Abbvie employs approximately 25,000 people worldwide and markets medicines in more than 170 countries.

In California, in September 2014, **Abbvie and Calico** announced a new partnership designed to synergies between the two companies with the aim to discover, develop and bring to market new therapies for patients suffering from age-related diseases, neurodegeneration and cancer.

Under the agreement, the companies will join forces to accelerate the availability of **new therapies** for age-related diseases: Calico will use its scientific expertise to build a research and development center in the world, with particular attention to the discovery and development of new and innovative drugs. Abbvie will provide support for such scientific and clinical development and its commercial experience to bring new discoveries to market. In September 2014 it was announced that Calico, in collaboration with Abbvie, has opened a research and development laboratory focused on aging and related diseases such as neurodegeneration and cancer. Initially, both companies will invest $ 250 million, with the possibility of investing a further 500 million. Calico will be responsible for research and development in the first five years and will continue to advance collaborative projects in Phase 2a for a period of ten years. The parties will equally share costs and profits.

On October 3, 2014, **President Obama** appointed Arthur D. Levinson, Founder and Chief Executive Officer of Calico, as one of eight recipients of the National Medal of Technology and Innovation. The award IS the highest honors from the nation to success and leadership in science and technology.

Levinson, a molecular biologist, has conducted pioneering work in genetics and biochemistry of cancer, and has contributed to the creation of personalized cancer therapies. Author or co-author of over 80 scientific papers and holder of 11 patents in the United States, he has won numerous awards for scientific and technological merit and in 2008 was elected a member of the American Academy of Arts and Sciences.

On March 24st, 2015 Ca.li.co. announced a four-year partnership with **QB3** also with the aim of improving the understanding of the biology of aging and potential **therapies** for age-related diseases.

QB3 is born from the cooperation between private industries and more than **250 scientists** from UC (California University) San Francisco, UC Berkeley and UC Santa Cruz. QB3 provides the UC research with the creation of mutually beneficial partnerships with industry and support entrepreneurs. The effort led to the launch of hundreds of biotech start-ups and significant job creation in the San Francisco Bay Area.

The partnership has **two sinergic components**: a research agreement to enable collaboration between Ca.li.co. and multiple QB3 workshops on specific programs related to aging, and a system of grants to support innovation in research on longevity led by QB3.

Expressing his gratitude to Calico, **Regis Kelly, director of QB3**, argues that addressing aging requires a translational perspective and multidisciplinary approach, towards which QB3 is precisely oriented.

Furthermore, on April 28st, 2015 Ca.li.co. and the **Buck Institute for Research** on aging have announced a collaboration-financial terms were not disclosed. the Buck Institute is the first independent organization in the United States and around the world dedicated to Neuroscience research for the study of the link between aging and chronic diseases. Headquartered in Novato, CA with 21 independent laboratories, the Buck institute is dedicated to extending the "healthspan" -years of healthy life- by slowing down the aging process. The Buck scientists work in collaboration with the laboratories that study mechanisms of aging and focus on prevention and treatment of age-related diseases such as Alzheimer's and Parkinson's, cancer, cardiovascular disease, macular degeneration, osteoporosis, diabetes and stroke.

Follow the latest developments in genomics, proteomics, bioinformatics and stem cell technologies[84].

".. This new partnership with Ca.Li.Co. is a unique way for university researchers and the biotechnology industry to work together in the field of aging," said Brian K. Kennedy, PhD, President and **Delegated Administrator** of the Buck Institute.

On July 21st, 2015 **AncestryDNA**, a leader in the field of genetics, and Ca.li.co., have announced a research project to investigate the hereditary aspect of the life span. They will evaluate anonymous data from millions of public family trees and a growing database of over a million genetic samples. Financial terms were not disclosed. AncestryDNA and Ca.li.co. will investigate the role of genetics and its influences in particularly longevity families using the database of ancestors and their algorithms. Ca.li.co. will therefore focus on the development and commercialization of potential therapies that emerge from the analysis. The research period will serve to identify common models of longevity by analyzing transmission through inheritance.

"Our common experience suggests that there may be hereditary factors behind longevity, but finding the genes responsible using standard techniques has proven elusive," said David Botstein, **Chief Scientific Officer of Ca.Li.Co.** and member of the National Academy of Sciences. "It is an extraordinary opportunity to address a fundamental unanswered question to the search for longevity with human pedigrees."[85]

Another examples of innovation towards the Commons models, in this case in the world of research, are the **American Gut Project** and the Hearth Microbiome Project. Such projects started in 2012 in California on the study of the intestinal bacterial population and its important implications in physiology and pathophysiology of many functions and alterations that underlie many diseases which affect not only the gastrointestinal tract but many organs in our body.

---

84 www.thebuck.org, last access 27.08.2015
85 http://www.calicolabs.com/news/2015/07/21/, last access 27.08.2015

This project involves a large population, co-opted into the project as a patient/investor with a **crowdfunding** financing structure. Each patient who participates invests € 99.00 giving its willingness to research and makes available its microbiota (intestinal bacteria collected through fecal examination) for a large scale study of the bacterial population and consequent individual mapping. The patient also benefits from a real blight monitoring, as well as any re-balancing therapies, or information preventive nature, valuable for one's health.

Prevention, useful for the patient after the mapping of intestinal bacteria may direct a significant number of diseases:

- oral cavity, stomach, duodenum (ulcers) and intestines (colitis and bowel diseases)
- obesity.

The American Gut is the largest research project funded through crowdfunding in 2012, now with **thousands of members**. All data obtained shall be made public within the limits of respect for privacy so that researchers and individuals can freely investigate, allowing anyone to establish new and interesting collaborations to be explored in more rigorous controlled trials. The project is open to participants of all nationalities[86].

---

86 Rob Knight Segui la pancia, non tutti i microbi vengono per nuocere, Rizzoli, ISBN 978-88-17-08196-2

7. New communication frontiers in health
Angelo Barbato

7.1 Fitness bracelets and wearable devices

Consumer electronics will see in 2015 an estimate of achievement of the possession of global smartphone 1.5 billion[87]. The **smartphone** will assume more the role of operational center in the connection of all the other useful items for everyday life and human health, which is the most important aspect of any action.

They are therefore increasingly developing more permanent connection with a growing number of objects (**Internet of Things**) network. Today, in addition to smartphone, the best-selling devices are: mobile standard, personal laptops, desktop personal computers, tablets, digital cameras and LCD TVs in total some 80% of consumer electronics. Small differences are found in developing countries, middle east, africa, china and india where 7 devices listed together represent about 64% of consumer electronics.

The Internet of Things will develop more and more will develop through the connection of sensors in **wearable devices** classified into two categories, the smartwatch and fitness devices.

A **smartwatch,** is a watch with additional features to the simple clock timing function.

Currently, we are in an embryonic stage in the development of **wearable devices** with a jumble of ideas that will select the most useful and high performance in environments increasingly internet of things. This will lead to an increasingly used virtual environments which will revolutionize also training and edu-

---

87 Enrico Pagliarini Radio 24 - 2024 del 9 gennaio 2015

cation.

The key feature that will see an exponential growth of these wearable electronic devices is represented by the **easy usage** that will allow a massive new growth in the world market which will start in more developed countries and will develop very quickly in emerging markets.

The exponential development of these devices will be driven by two key elements: the **sensors** of all kinds that are developing and the tendency towards **permanent connection** through Wifi or 4G.

The world organization of telecommunications began the process of standardization of **5G**. It will arrive in 2020 and will ensure the connection of up to 1 million units / km² for the development of Internet of things with a bandwidth capacity of up to 20 GB.

Every three months, Akamai publishes a report on the state of the internet[88] that illustrates the performance of the network around the world. Measurements performed by Akamai are reliable, since it represents the largest company specializing in the distribution of content in the world (**content delivery network**). This type of company offers its' own consultancy for the speeding up of the content display.

Akamai has a network of about 170,000 servers in a hundred countries around the world and thus enables to load pages faster on the internet or view videos. For this reason, content delivery networks are well aware of the conditions of the network in the world. **Asia** is the continent where optical fiber is the most developed. Ireland leads the way in Europe with 17.4 Mb / sec.

The Italian government approved the decree on 03/03/2015 regarding optical fiber, postponing the implementation at a later decision of the CIPE- Interministerial Committee for Economic Planning. Telecom Italia is currently the company with the highest turnover (Fastweb is the second), still with much of

---

88 Enrico Pagliarini Radio 24 - 2024 del 26 giugno 2015

its infrastructure in copper. The issue of geographical network is such an important infrastructure that the President of the Council, **Matteo Renzi,** wrote in his program that he would serve a public network society. Obviously we need optical fiber because companies must invest in technology that has connectivity as a stronghold through the internet of things. There is no use in mentioning cloud or the internet of things without **connectivity**.

The latest report from Akamai puts **Italy** is in 56th place for the average speed of the connection in the world with 5.6 Mb / sec.

The sensors will be developed mainly in the following disciplines: **health, fitness** and sports, home automation (**smarthome** for switches and lighting), energy, mobility and sharing economy.

The **sensors** are defined as *transducers,* in direct interaction with the measured system. Such devices are born historically to display the physical quantities in a simple and immediate way.

With the *development of electronics* sensors have had a considerable **expansion** that will increase further with the internet of things especially in medicine, in industry, in robotics and in general in all control systems.

Sensors are becoming ever more powerful at decreasing costs. They basically they consist of: **physical and chemical sensors**. The sensors are of **image, motion, alarm (safety** such as smoke detectors), of **pressure** (to detect the expectations), of **voice** (microphone), **humidity, temperature (thermostats), ultraviolet** (for measuring the emission radiation), and more.

Among the **motion** sensors will greatly develop:
- vehicle detector in the blind zone (overtaking);
- sensor for the maintenance of the lane;
- dynamic speed control that allows to keep the vehicle in a constant manner below a speed limit even without the control of the driver as in the case of abrupt braking of the car that precedes, objects suddenly crossing the road or distraction of the driver.

Development of the internet of things will increasingly see use of **smartphone** as a control center and sensors such as network nodes.

In biology the **sense organs** can be considered living beings' sensors. Man interacts with the outside world through the five senses (smell, sight, hearing, touch, taste), cats whiskers are kind of sensors of touch and proximity, in the internet of things objects interact with the outside world through sensors and communicate with each other through the network.

With wearable electronics it is possible via smartphone (ECU) to analyze the information coming from **wearable sensors** located in watches (smartwatch), fitness bracelets and sunglasses.

The fantasy of viable wearable devices will lead the **market** to produce more different devices such as toothbrushes with sensors that assess the effectiveness in cleaning the teeth (dental). Among them, the sensors can achieve any combination, used in applications for the smartphone or health and those who have greater impetus will be the ones useful for monitoring the state of health and prevention in different environments: Domestic (homesmart) and mobile environments (car, train, airplane, etc.) and used to save energy.

The **communication protocols** and **energy consumption** will be the key for the exponential growth of the internet of things which will need the establishment of guidelines to allow their tidy, efficient and effective utilization. For now there are a lot of ideas but they must mature for an appropriate exponential growth.

Many products are whims often linked to **fashion** and designers and sometimes you do not understand what expensive smartwatches or fitness bracelets (about 300 Euros) with functions overlapping the smartphone, are even for. Sometimes more more than real consumer needs these are real attempts to invoice the seller.

In the future development, the secret of success will be

trying to make these **truly useful** devices: will they improve or change my life? Do they make life easier? They are developing a lot of opportunities for the future but they are still first-generation devices with the limits of the immaturity of the market beginnings.

The challenge is open especially in the field of **energy** of the **transportation** of such devices with the use of current batteries that need replacement batteries because the technological innovation that is able to extend decisively their duration has not yet developed.

The revolution also involves the **health sector** as well as relating to the energy (with safeguarding through prevention the healthy individual as long as possible), the communication (via the internet of things) and logistics (through new models of taking charge of individuals) will see an exponential development also as regards the production of medical devices.

The latter will see an exponential growth thanks to increasing use of **3D printers** that will increasingly have a central role in the development of the internet of things.

China has already seen the **first surgery** that allowed the reconstruction of a spinal implant in a young patient with spinal malformation.

There is a specialization of medicine that deals with accidents and injuries in the work area, or **occupational health**.

There is a specialization of medicine then that deals with the prevention of disease not only in workplaces and in job opportunities but expanding its principles to disease prevention in a holistic way by analyzing the environmental causes localized in pollutants in air, water and soil. This specialization is called **hygiene and preventive medicine**.

Therefore, prevention also means using systems that through the sensors can **avoid accidents and injuries**. Just think of the anti-collision systems or automatic parking through the use of unmanned mobile vehicles (cars, trains, planes etc.), Fundamental systems in congested areas such as large metropolitan areas (Beijing, Shanghai in China). These technologies applied to the internet of things will have an exponential growth.

Installers, be they doctors or technicians will have to adapt to this exponential growth of devices that will revolutionize the well-being and prevention of diseases and accidents. In the contrary case it will be the market to increase the development of self-installing devices.

Many of these devices will have a very long **battery** life (up to years), related to renewable energies (rechargeable, solar, mechanical, etc.). It will connect to Wi-Fi internet and create a network of things starting from the house.

Already today many companies in the United States require internet access to **home thermometer** and based on the cost of energy and on the outside weather conditions (summer/winter/day/night) they can intervene on on the climate of the house and the consequent environmental well-being, energetic and economic health of the environment.

7.2 Telemedicine

Telemedicine is the provision of information and health services via **telecommunications technologies.**

Telehealth is a **broad definition** that includes basic services, such as two health professionals discussing a case over the phone or how to do more complex robotic surgery between implants in different areas of the globe.

Originally used for administrative functions or health education, telemedicine today highlights a **myriad of technological solutions**.

For example, doctors use **e-mail** for prescription drugs and to provide other health services.

The most significant use of telemedicine is now **home monitoring conditions** of the clinical condition of the patients, whose clinical trial in the UK has shown improvements in the mortality of about 47%.

Monitoring biometrics data

Using your smartphone, you can centrally monitor many **biometric data**: blood pressure, heart rate, weight, distance traveled, time waking sleep. Prolonged monitoring overcomes the single data, accurate and to make sustained aggregate analysis over time and may even allow the possibility of the contact card link with their healthcare provider or facility. In this way, the smartphone itself also becomes a powerful prevention tool.

Qardio is a company operating in the United States founded by Italians [89](Marco Peluso is Chief Executive Officer) that develops products and services through app monitoring for medical guidance. Apps are of 3 types: Quardio arm to monitor blood pressure, Quardio basis for monitoring weight and Quardio heart for ECG monitoring and dynamic holter through a wearable

89 Enrico Pagliarini Radio 24 - 2024 del 27 marzo 2015

device. These devices collect statistics with advantages in monitoring with diagnostic value for both the general practitioner as well as for the Medical Specialist Cardiologist.

New Communication promotes the patient doctor/relationship with an approach more closely geared towards the patient. For example, **Quardio heart** beyond the ECG tracing that shows the heart rate, also records tracked temperature and physical activity, the doctor is so favored in the diagnosis of arrhythmia as it is possible to be monitored for 365 days a year. The application allows the doctor then, through software algorithms, to monitor hundreds of patients in real time.

8. Health care orientated by the patient
Bruno Corda, Angelo Barbato

As reiterated in several other parts of this book, we are living an epochal transition from the capitalist economy to the economy of **commons**.

This exciting phase of transformation between vertical and hierarchical relations that are constantly undermined by new emerging horizontal and distributed models is increasing exponentially both in relation to the world of **production** as for **services**.

No **service** may be much closer to the collaborative and participatory dimension of the commons than **healthcare**.

The health service is definitely the **most important** service, as it touches the most personal sphere of the life of individuals, sharing of medical data, leads commons into the most intimate sphere, data on personal health and on energy parameters (healthy individuals) , data on personal parameters for the energy deficit (sick people), and on in the synthesis of life and death of each of us.

Health care, centered in the fundamental paradigm of the **doctor/patient relationship**, traditionally a vertical and closed relationship reserved between doctor and patient in which the first gives prescriptions and the second passively follows accordingly, was suddenly transformed into a distributed, equal and horizontal relationship.

Throughout healthcare history it has been crucial even before the treatment, the relationship that develops between doctor and patient. The innovation we are witnessing is the transformation from the rigid verticality of that relationship, in a new system of **circular confrontation**, continuous and open, involving mutually patients, doctors, researchers, technicians with the aim of improving the care provided to the patient and general health of society. This new circular movement of information becomes a fundamental basis also and especially for prevention.

The innovation in this open system where information exchange takes place in a horizontal manner between patients, doctors, researchers and other individuals interested in the world of health has developed **spontaneously** as a result of the fact that more and more people have started to search the internet for explanations on their symptoms to have an accurate picture of their medical condition.

This happened starting those who had already been diagnosed and began to tell the story of their own disease or disorder, hoping to receive **feedback** from people with a similar story.

The **democratization of health** has also allowed others, unsatisfied with the therapeutic solutions prescribed by their doctor, to start to search the web for people with similar concerns, hoping to have news of alternative treatments. With the development of distributed systems of communication through the Internet the limitation due to autoreferentiality, inherent in the doctor-patient vertical relationship, has been **overcome**. This has produced benefits not only for the patient who has come to have more awareness, more information and more possibilities of alternative therapeutic pathways but also for the doctor and for researchers who see widening the discussion and the possibilities of new information and the opening of references. The result is an exponential enrichment for all through a **circular system** that produces new benefits to the patient as is the principle of circular quality theory.

With increasing life expectancy and the consequent increase of one or more chronic conditions, more and more people undergoing **treatment at times perceived by the patient inadequate or insufficient** or even excessive began to organize themselves together to seek **new therapies.**

In the vertical style doctor/ patient relationship, where the patient passively follows the prescription of medication without the possibility of participation, the issue of **adherence to therapy** has inevitably emerged over time. Adherence is the extent to which the patient follows the recommendations made by the team of health care, which the patient has accepted after receiving detailed information about it[90].

Failure to comply can be classified into two broad categories: **intentional and unintentional.**

When the failed adhesion of the therapy is **intentional,** it is characterized by a patient's conscious choice to not take the therapy. This attitude can have rational or irrational aspects. In the first case this position is due to the subjective belief that:

- the medicines are not effective,

- the medicaments can be potentially toxic,

- there is direct or indirect cost problems for the prescribed therapy.

The **unintentional non-adhesion** can also be irrational, as an emotional response to the disease and therapy. Intentional forms lead to the making of a partial treatment or even the discontinuation of treatment.

In **unintentional nonadherence** to therapy, the patient has an explicit willingness to follow treatment but has difficulties in doing so. This problem is due to external reasons, extremely variable and largely related to the socio-economic context. Also part of this category the so-called "forgotten" and "jump" of the dose[91].

On the Internet there are already several models of open source **health commons** involving collaboratively doctors, patients, researchers and technicians. These collaborative platforms were essential in the process of empowerment of patients and in the circulation of information. Differently from the initial mistrust, these tools have not brought a disconnection between doc-

---

90 M Fliedner, RN, MSN, Sabine Degen Kellerhals, RN, Erik Aerts, RN, Aderenza alle terapie farmacologiche anti-tumorali per via orale, 2013 EBMT
91 F Colivicchi et al - Aderenza terapeutica, G Ital Cardiol Vol 11 Suppl 3 al n 5 2010

tor and patient but created synergies by adding value.

The most active patients have organized in non-profit groups constituted especially for rare diseases; these are more or less organized, with different objectives: **practical and psychological support, public awareness towards the diseases, demand for greater public investment in search.**

In the collaborative health commons, online interactive information exchange models represent an **advantage** for both **patients** and their **doctors and researchers.**

Even the Americans **epidemiologists** currently recognize the usefulness of online circular information as complementary or supplementary to the Monitoring validated models used in traditional research.

Online information is to be particularly valuable in the reporting **side effects** of drugs, significantly underestimated in traditional collection systems.

The number of people who **share** data on their health and your medical conditions is growing exponentially.

This information is also a source usable by **research programs**. The new approach to research is based on crowdsourcing. Crowdsourcing, a creation model or development of a project object or idea of an indefinite set of people not previously organized. This process is encouraged by the tools that are made available on the web. Usually the call of the open mechanism is made available through the portals present on the Internet[92].

The **crowdsourcing** model is radically different from the method of randomized controlled trials typical of traditional research, costly in terms of time and money, organized and led from the top, relegating patients to the role of passive subjects. Frank Moss, director of the MIT Media Lab, an interdisciplinary research laboratory at the Massachusetts Institute of Technology dedicated to projects at the convergence of technology, multimedia, science, art and design; says that "In fact we transform pa-

---

92 https://it.wikipedia.org/wiki/Crowdsourcing last access 17.09.2015

tients into scientists, changing the balance of forces among clinicians, scientists and patients. "

The new, more spacious **sanitary commons** are transforming the medical sector, both from a theoretical setting point of view and from that of the operating practice.

Among the most popular s**ocial media sites** we find **PatientsLikeMe, ACOR, the Lam Foundation, Treatments Together, the Life Raft Group, the Organization for Autism Research, Chordoma Foundation and LmSarcoma Direct Research**.

Many health care patient-oriented sites are the result of personal stories, often related to **rare diseases** that received little attention and even less commitment to finding therapeutic solutions.

The Association of Cancer Online Resources (**ACOR**)[93], founded by Gilles Frydman, did make a further step in the concept of patient-oriented health care, creating greater health commons that engages more than 600,000 people between patients and therapists in 163 public communities online.

Already in some innovative platforms patients report about their own situation and **researchers** develop protocols, in ACOR, however, **patients** share scientific information to therapists, **operating jointly** with in the organization of new data collection and aggregation methods, aimed to address research on their diseases. "

Patients are also dedicated to raising money for scientific research. These patients online, the **e-patients**, are giving birth to what Frydman called a "participatory medicine" model, where a single commons various subjects converge: patients, researchers, doctors, financiers, manufacturers of medical equipment, therapists, pharmaceutical companies and healthcare professionals, all committed to work together to improve patient care.

The new models of sharing (Commons) health also come

---

93 http://www.acor.org/ , last access 19.09.2015

to **modify** the traditional way of **funding research**.

The **classical funding.** in fact are born of ideas originated by researchers, favoring targeted research excellence, effect, high impact and visibility, capable of creating networks able to finance young researchers, favoring large chapters such as inflammation, immunology, vaccines and often leaving the researchers to start work and only later seek funding classics.

The **patient-oriented research** is aimed instead "on demand" to give answers to specific questions that start from the interests of patients and not of the researchers, looking at results and not at the publications and impact factor. In addition, it may comprise very different themes from the traditional hierarchical search, and it can be used as substrate for future classic research.

PatientsLikeMe, a network for health care addressed to more than 200,000 patients, who treat over 1800 diseases, published the first observational study initiated by patients who either failed to rebut the conclusions of a conventional research, according to which drugs based on lithium carbonate could arrest the neurodegenerative progress of amyotrophic lateral sclerosis (ALS). The organization announced that it had "developed a new algorithm designed to compare the data of patients who reported taking lithium with other ALS patients who showed a trend of similar illness." Following 348 patients who were using lithium "**off-label**", PatientsLikeMe found that "the lithium had no observable effect on the evolution of the disease in those patients."

Although the direct verification by patients via online platforms can not hold a candle to a controlled clinical, double-blinded trial; it does hpñd the advantage of being faster and with reduced costs, representing a new, efficient search tool.

One of the great advantages of patient-oriented research is its speed, thanks to which we can get valuable information more quickly than professional researchers, forced to make a long series of steps that will last a long **time**, up to decades. The professional search structurally requires a long standby time, that constitutes the difference between the time at which an important medical discovery is known by some people, and the moment in which is communicated to all.

Additionally, **controlled clinical studies**, double-blind, are extremely expensive, while **observational studies** initiated by patients using **big data** and algorithms to identify health patterns and developments can be undertaken at a marginal cost approaching zero.

The **open source approach to research** is still in its infancy, and lies often at that stage of verification that the slow process of professional research, with its testing over time, provides for controlled randomized studies. Supporters of the led by patients' research are well aware of these shortcomings, but they are also convinced that this new reality will have an appropriate verification system, similar to Wikipedia introducing control mechanisms, review and confirmation of its entries. Wikipedia now has 19 million employees ; thousands of users carry out checks and improve the articles, making the level of accuracy of this open source portal comparable to that of other encyclopedias. Today, Wikipedia is the eighth most visited site in the world, and is an encyclopedia of universal knowledge with millions of contacts. Thinking about the health commons oriented by patients, we are thrown back to the early days of online Wikipedia, when the academic community sentenced the democratization of research would seriously compromise the high scientific standards, required by the compilation of an encyclopedia. Fears proved unfounded, and the supporters of open source health commons oriented by patients wonder why research crowdsourcing, when it is informed of strict scientific protocols, should show worse results.

9. The democratization of health
Bruno Corda, Angelo Barbato

Doctors who use the network to exchange information and experiences with patients and other physicians, comparing therapeutic solutions and new models of interpretation of diagnostic utilities, especially for those diseases not yet well classified, is constantly increasing. **Dan Hoch,** a neurologist at Massachusetts General Hospital who specializes in treating epilepsy through e-patients, realized that the traditional vertical and taboos in patients continuing involvement resulted highly anachronistic, especially for chronic conditions and great complexity[94].

Another colleague, neurologist at Massachusetts General Hospital, **John Lester** has even set up an online community that brought together over 300 grassroots groups, who treated online a number of neurological diseases, including Alzheimer's, multiple sclerosis, Parkinson's disease, Huntington's disease and epilepsy. Such site is regularly consulted by over 200,000 people all over the world.

Today, the Internet has hundreds of open source **health commons** and their number will increase significantly in the coming years.

It has surprisingly been observed that only **30%** of the online commons interventions was oriented on **moral support** while the remaining **70%** had as its objective the search for better **therapeutic solutions**, both in the management of the protocols, observation and limiting the side effects and on how to deal with the disease on a daily basis. The information exchanged allowed to deepen the preparation not only superior to that of the

---

94 Dan Hoch e Tom Ferguson, What I've Learned from e-patients, in "PLOS Medicine",2,8,2005, http://journals.plos.org/plosmedicine/article?id=10.1371/journal.pmed.0020206, last access 21.09.2015

number of participating patients, but also, at least in terms of amplitude, to that of many doctors, even specialists in the field.

Hoch saw the importance of the knowledge of the emerging empirical data from individual experiences of patients, which although not members of an epidemiological model previously established, had two great advantages: numerosity and extreme speed of acquisition. The **scientific observation path** is this **reversed**. Emerging data are evaluated and processed according to scientific criteria of selection that significantly reduce the bias (error) os selection.

This reversed process diverging from traditional studies has the advantage of being **fast** and very **economical**. Flanked with traditional studies, this may represent a synergistic contribution of great impact in the knowledge of many diseases are still not clearly understood.

The **Health IT Summit**, which was held in **San Francisco** between the 3rd and 4th of March 2015, was made of the situation on big data for domestic use. It emerged that results are still shy to overcome the resistance represented by the use of very different technologies to each other and consequently with difficulties of dialogue and interface.

Dr. Kaelber of Metro Health has estimated that the health system will be able to enhance the analysis of data only from **2040**[95].

In 2009, the US government has allocated 1 billion and 200 million dollars to help healthcare facilities to acquire stock electronic. The **big data** that will therefore generate in the United States and other countries, will form a pool of information that, if properly exploited by open source health commons oriented by patients, may, subject to the necessary guarantees of confidentiality, revolutionize the the health sector by making services in assistance to the sick more efficient.

---

95 Dan Verel http://medcitynews.com/2015/03/will-data-analytics-health-care-take-2040-fully-realized-highlights-health-summit/, last access 26.09.2015

The big data in health,during the winter of 2013, were invaluable when a serious **flu epidemic** worldwide spread rapidly. Following the data of online research on issues related to influenza, google was able to identify the hatcheries of the disease and the intensity with which it manifested, and follow the spreading in real time. Obviously, the analysis is not as simple as it appears, Google had overestimated the intensity of the epidemic, also due to excessive alarmism of media (especially social media), from which many people had been induced to seek information on the influenza. Despite the overestimation, the detections made by Google turned out so reliable as **to induce the centers for Disease control and prevention** in the US to **officially involve the company** in their monitoring programs.

The use of the internet during an **epidemic** allows the chance to follow in real time the spread of infection. This is critical to keep the disease under control (surveillance) for quickly alerting local health departments to prepare the timely administration of the vaccines.

Once again, Internet proves to be unbeatable in the paradigm of communication and speed of the intercepting the **earliest reactions to the epidemic**, when people, often several days before calling your doctor or go to be examined, conduct research on the web to see if the their symptoms match those of the disease. With the **traditional monitoring system**, the data collection takes one or two **weeks** for doctors to visit the sick in the various parts of a country: excessive time because a virus can reach the widest possible dissemination or even finish his journey in such a span.

The power of the speed of the communication paradigm is not only represented by google, **twitter** also could prove a valuable monitoring tool considering that users of social networks exchange every day 500 million messages.

For now, the institutional centers of Public Health show that these early warning **tools** play a secondary role until at times becoming **complementary** with institutional surveillance systems. Perfecting the algorithms so as to exclude interferences and achieving an accurate data reading can make google and twitter tools for monitoring and detection, potentially representing supervision centers and containment of epidemics using big data. Fighting the contagion will **save billions of dollars in health care costs**, providing a monitoring and tracking system that will increasingly marginal costs close to zero.

Organ transplants are among the most expensive medical applications, but also on these grounds, thanks to new discoveries, the potential of reducing costs significantly is not too far away. Soon, in fact, tissues and organs needed for a transplant will be produced with a **3D printing** process, once again at modest marginal costs, or close to zero. The three-dimensional printing of parts of the human body is already well advanced. Using living cells, the **Wake Forest Institute for Regenerative Medicine, in North Carolina**, has recently printed a prototype of a **human kidney** with a 3D bioprinting process. Organovo, a biotech company based in San Diego, has created functioning human liver tissues. Researchers at the ARC Centre of Excellence for electromaterials Science of the University of Wollongong, Australia, are experimenting with the use of 3D printing processes to produce living cells of the muscle and nervous tissue. Cameron Ferris, a researcher of the institute explains: "The technology we use is the same as the inkjet printers, but instead of ink we use various types of cells." Playing living tissue from the body cells of a patient, instead of implanting the organ from a donor, avoids problems of rejection.

It is expected that in the next ten years, the **3D bioprinting of organic tissue** - cardiac and nerve tissue, blood vessel segments, cartilage Impaired joints, etc. - Will become common. To get to bioprint whole organs we must instead wait a bit longer.

Stuart Williams, a researcher at the **institute of cardiovascular innovation Louisville, Kentucky**, is conducting experiments with cells from fat extracted by liposuction: it would mix them with glue and then proceed to the printing of a heart. Williams believes that it will be possible to get to the **3D printing of a 'bio-ficial " heart within a decade.**

Gordon Wallace, at the aRc center, argues that "by **2025** we will probably be able to **produce fully functioning organs**, manufactured tailored to each individual patient," probably within a few decades the new frontier of 3D bioprinting of replacement parts for the human body will be conquered. As for the other forms of molding in 3D, with the progress of technology the production costs of these biological substitutes will decrease.

In a society of big data and marginal costs almost zero, the **current, enormous health care costs** (not rarely rudimentary, scarcely updated and wasteful) will be a **thing of the past.**

After the democratization of information through the internet, electricity democratization through the internet of energy, the democratization of production through the open source 3D printing, the democratization of higher education through Mooc and democratization through the economy of participation, the potential **health care democratization through the web** also adds to the social economy, making the collaborative commons a force able to affect the life of society even more deeply.

10. The new community care in Italian public
Antonio Magi

Development processes of the health care systems of Western countries are characterized by numerous factors of **instability** that can be traced back to the development of pathologies to which health systems must respond.

We must not forget the evolution of some social phenomena linked to the **healthcare consumerism** on one side, and on the other **defensive medicine** that pushes towards higher diagnostic tests on the other that have triggered an increase in demand and cost of health care systems. This spiral has undermined the fragile balance between social spending and taxation by activating a strong demand for change.

We must not underestimate the fact that from the analysis of health systems, often due to the **bureaucratization** of work processes to the point of increased dissatisfaction of patients commonly linked to the standby time, the emergence of strong inequalities of health and use of health services; we are faced with major changes in the process of acquiring and disseminating knowledge about health problems which has undergone a process of profound transformation thanks to the internet.

These changes alter the traditional relationship of power that governs the **doctor-patient relationship.**

The stages of change

The health systems of Western countries are affected by at least three phases:

- A **first phase** characterized by separation and **competition** where the cultural facility assumed that the dynamics of competition were able to steer the production of public goods and not only private ones.

Starting from this setting a reformer path has stepped forward and sought to bring the culture and the **typical production**

processes of manufacturing enterprises or production facilities of private goods to health services.

In this regard there are **those who still claim** that even in the healthcare sector, the reform program was aimed to introduce the typical mechanisms of the market and to develop competition.

The goal of increasing efficiency and competition among the various components of the health system has been prosecuted following different strategies, created in different ways among the **various national governments.**

These reforming processes, however, have not produced the expected efficiency results and the introduction of competition has not curbed the increase in health systems costs, indeed, the dynamics of competition have highlighted the difficulty of adjusting production processes.

- A **second step** was oriented on integration and control with the attempt to solve the problems of public regulation by shifting the axis on market dynamics and competition that had given rise to other critical factors.

It has been shown that the widespread **privatization** and the adoption of a purely market logic in the management of welfare services had presented four sets of issues. A territorial distribution of providers (private and nonprofit) became disconnected from the expression of need; the risk occurred of producing a loss of identity in the nonprofit (risk of isomorphic behavior towards the private profit); as well as the delegitimization of the state's function by undermining its role as actor in the redistributive processes and guarantee against the risk of social disintegration; therefore finally an increase in social inequalities.

In fact, economic studies have highlighted **the lack of efficiency of competitive dynamics** (at least when this becomes a unique strategy to regulate the system) in the systems of control that govern the production of public goods, concluding that the introduction of market principles and corporatization in the management of health services showed the need to experiment with other ways, able to take into account the specific nature of health systems.

These critical elements and the debate that ensued have just started the second phase of change. Moving towards a direction opposite to the one introduced by the first wave (of change), some governments have preferred to force the role of private providers, reducing (or officially only in practice), the freedom of choice provided for patients. Also, in some states such as France, Britain and New Zealand, there has been **increase** in the local **public authority power** to plan and regulate health care and introduction of new bonds and controls in the practice of medicine.

Even these processes, aimed at seeking a **rebalance between the dynamics of the market and those of public regulation**, have taken different forms in each country, in relation to the specific dynamics of the territorial contexts (social actors, perhaps policies, their roles and vindicating capacity etc.).

Result: **health spending has continued to grow** and to affect more and more on the gross domestic product of individual states. On the other hand the possibility of citizens' choice has been limited and in most countries the citizens have expressed dissatisfaction with the functioning of health services.

These elements have caused the loss of driving force of the slogans that had characterized the previous period. The tension towards privatization and market loses standing and guidelines pave its way to draw the attention of decision makers towards a further stage.

- A **third phase** is focused on the **quality of services** and patients' rights. The reforms undertaken in the period from the end of last century to the early years of the new, in countries such as the Netherlands, New Zealand, Sweden, France and Germany, offered some basic rights which rethink the services of welfare. In particular, they recognized the right to receive adequate information about the state of health and possible treatment options, to have access to their health data, to be treated with dignity, to have respect for their privacy, to get a second option about their diagnosis, to express their grievances, while not having to wait too long.

The analysis of this long process of reform, which accompanied the health systems of Western countries, highlights the intake of **different characteristics**, in times and forms. For another, it is difficult to identify the precise effect of the different factors that have influenced these changing dynamics.

We can only retrieve a list of elements that various researches indicate as generative factors of **welfare policies**. The socio-economic structure of the countries, the political system, the cultural matrix that guides the behavior and assertive capacities of different actors (professionals, citizens, policy makers), the features and the strategic behavior of the third sector and profit enterprises, are all factors which help to define the guidelines that have influenced the reform process.

The reinterpretation of the change process also allows to see that it is an endogenous change aimed at increasing the efficiency of the system as a whole and that, as such, **never takes the form of structural change**.

What is emerging on the horizon of the health systems in individual countries is a **change of pace** of the reforming process, the changes enabled or being implemented have a good break with the reformist path of the recent years.

Structural change: towards community care

By analyzing current reform processes, one can easily notice that the keywords refer to a **shift** of the center of the process of care **from the hospital to the territorial zone**, and that the most evoked keywords in the debate and the regulatory tools refer to primary care.

The debates and ongoing experiences show that these terms underlie (and evoke) a **paradigm shift**, around which the processes and dynamics of the care are being redefined. Rethinking of a new paradigm of care with regards to Community Care is now less difficult than in the past.

In this perspective we can imagine that innovation must be analyzed relating to **doctor-patient dynamics**, to those between different professionals and finally to those with other community actors. The specification of these three directions of innovation push to adopt the term **Community Care** as a reference capable of representing the complexity of the directions that need to be considered.

Today we propose to consider: "the **user-centered** care work" as the amount of change in the relationship between those who provide and those who receive the benefit; "**Teamwork**" as the way forward to change the relationships between professionals; and "n**etwork governance**" as a governance process of the dynamics with and within the communities.

Primary care and innovation

	Social Innovation	Technological Innovation
Doctor-patient relationship (involvement in the path of cure)	• CARE WORK CENTRALIZED ON THE PATIENT with an holistic approach • Professional identity and balanced Evidence based Medicine with Narrative Based Medicine • Empowerment	• Electronic health care card • social network
Relation among MMG-PLS-Specialists Territorial professionals, other healthcare opera-	COORDINATION AND PROFESSIONAL INTEGRATION (Horizontal and vertical)	• Shared healthcare file • social network

tors and integration with the hospital	• Identity and professional integration • teamwork • Timeline management	• e-research method
Relation with (and for) the community	COMMUNITY • Integration of policies • Promotion of health • Reduction of social inequalities • network governance	• social-network • e-democracy

At the conclusion of the definition of the patient-centered model, **five** fundamental aspects are proposed, linked to the need to:

- consider the **person as a whole**, paying attention to the biological, psychological and social dimensions;
- keep in mind that the patient is a **unique individual** with perceptions and ways to treat its disease condition;
- **share power and responsibilities**, with due attention to patient preferences and the need to exchange information and involve the patient in the process leading to the choice of treatment;
- pay attention to the construction of the **therapeutic alliance** relationship based on shared objectives to be pursued;
- keep in mind that **the doctor is a person**, influenced by professional practice but also by personal qualities and subjectivity.

When the doctor tries to apply the results of scientific research to the clinical case in front of him, a sort of **cognitive dissonance** is immediately created. Dissonance is produced by the inability to take into account the complexity and uniqueness of the individual.

The discrepancy between the clinical dimension addressed through the analysis of the symptoms and pursued through the interpretation of the individual parameters on a statistical basis, the systemic dimension of the functioning of the human body and the reworking of the subjective experience of the disease from the patient, requires a recomposition of **holistic kind**.

The complexity of this process is given by the presence of certain factors that affect the process of care, in particular we can talk about is a comparison between the **segmentation of clinical information** and the need to consider (and redefine its significance) in a **global perspective** the clinical comparison between data interpretation (objective and/ or subjective) made by the physician or by the patient in the light of her own experiences, which also contains emotional implications vs highly differentiated cognitive one.

These elements of complexity, revised in light of a patient-centered approach, highlight the need to build a treatment process that combines the "analytical" contribution of evidence (its culture of **Evidence Based Medicine**) with the "understanding" provided by reconstruction of the original features inherent in the personal stories (Narrative Based Medicine).

A further element of complexity is related to the choice, inherent in the logic of intervention centered on the user, assigning great importance to the processes of **communication** between those who provide and those who receive the health service.

The effectiveness of health care and health promotion processes depend on the ability to successfully resolve the ambiguities elements that characterize the **complex situation**.

The medical profession has built its identity and personal identification codes around a **specialist knowledge** that has found its highest expression in the development of systems within their region and that of the more specialized hospital.

This type of identity development and knowledge has led us to consider (by users, but also by health workers) territorial medical and hospital specialists, with regards to their logistics expertise, as bearers of the true knowledge; and the general territorial ones as organizational and **'bureaucratic'** handmaidens of the system. Such phenomena is trying to be reversed in italy by giving specialist skills to those who do not have any, instead of putting together the different generalist and specialist skills as a team for the common good of the patient/ user.

This surely simplistic representation of professional identities, in fact, has been challenged by the **Ottawa Charter**[96], which reaffirms the centrality of the territory and the need to integrate a specialized knowledge with a holistic one that considers the people as a whole. Until now this knowledge has been experienced by professionals, but also by users of the services, as hierarchically sequential, so we tend to think that the real knowledge is in the specialized hospital.

These cultural stereotypes end up creating the idea of professionals (doctors in particular) of **Series A and Series B**, where, of course, the series is represented by the specialized hospital. Another element that differentiates the professional cultures of health concerns the organizational context.

In **Italy**, on the one hand we talk about hospital doctors and other physicians who work in the territory (whether GPs, paediatricians PLS or outpatient specialists). In the first case of hospital doctors are referred to professionals who act as employees within complex organizational systems, while in the second of professionals accustomed to working alone (MMG and PLS) and, finally, quasi-subordinates working, instead within organizational and territorial systems, as employees (Specialists Outpatient).

---

96 https://it.wikipedia.org/wiki/Promozione_della_salute, last access 01.11.2015

Obviously organizational cultures and habits in the management of the professional everyday life are profoundly different for **general practitioners** and for **pediatricians**. The decision-making autonomy, the relationship with authority and power, the need for sharing and time organization are very different and, consequently, lead to development of various organizational skills. These different organizational cultures and professional identity have failed to developed over time integration capabilities, but rather mutual distrust and lack of legitimacy. The development of a territorial system can not ignore the mutual legitimacy of the professions in the field and the redefinition of an integrated knowledge, capable of synthesizing skills and of their assimilation.

Identity and Professions

	Ospedale	**Territorio**
Nature and knowledge	Specialist	Holistic
Professional Relations	Intra-professional (between specialized knowledge)	Interprofessional (between professions and organizations)
CulturE	Profession and organization	Profession

The keywords on which the central role of the territory in care work play are attributable to the legitimacy of a **holistic knowledge** to be able to integrate different knowledge and perspectives of professionals who may be involved.

We can talk about **integration** between professions (operational) with reference to the coercion practices of individual professionals who are acting in the same case.

The experiences of innovation relate to the integration between general practitioners and medical specialists working in the territory aggregated into functional structures (AFT **combinations Territorial Functional**); between general practitioners and local specialists who work in the territory and who manage the chronicity (Collaboration between AFT and AFT of MMG territorial Specialist) and doctors working in the hospital and involved (mainly) in the acute condition of the disease; among all doctors in the area (MMG-PLS-Territorial Specialists) with other health professions and health figures, in general, non health related but social, educational (etc.) involved in care work in the territory (UCCP Complex Units of Primary care) or hospitals (H).

The centrality of the **integration processes** and the need to rethink the paradigm that characterizes the health professions towards holistic logic is, moreover, very present in the innovation experiences of primary care services.

The reasons intrinsic to the care work are attributable to:

- the importance of exchange between primary care physicians and specialists regarding the patient's situation;
- the development of mentoring and teaching activities;
- the provision of prevention activities in relation to alcohol and smoking;
- prevention against obesity;
- involvement in care networks;
- the satisfaction of professional activity;
- work considered professionally rewarding;
- participation in professional evaluation practices.

But the elements that seem to better able to define the identity can be traced to the **integration activity among general practitioners and specialists**, and **prevention** activities. These two elements are certainly indicators of a change in focus that shifts the identity axis from specialization to integration of skills and attention to prevention. This shift towards the recomposition of knowledge does not, however, only regard the professional

160

identity, but also impacts organizational processes that guide the course of treatment. In this perspective it becomes the center of teamwork development.

Ultimately, from the point of view of patients, team work has many positive effects that reinforce the importance of considering this aspect as one of the basic elements of primary care. This analysis, supported by a fair review of the literature, leads to argue that **team** organization allows to produce:
- better health outcomes;
- shorter standby times;
- a better quality of care;
- a greater degree of customer empowerment;
- increased user satisfaction;
- a reduction in visits to doctors;
- less hospitalization;
- less use of medicaments for the patient;
- an increase in the delivery of preventive care;
- healthier behaviors;
- increased frequency of early diagnosis.

In studies undertaken in the **United Kingdom, Australia and Canada**, on the activity of primary care; physicians report that the group work together with other medical specialists and non-medical professionals, produces a better ability to manage certain chronic diseases (eg diabetes, asthma management, hypertension etc.).

The basis of these researches are signaled to be the effects of **shared responsibility**, attention to the totality of the person and increased attention to prevention.

The mechanisms that lead to **better results** in terms of outcome can be traced to the fact that:
- the presence of different professionals allows you to distribute work among all the members of the group. In particular, this frees doctors from the organizational burden and from work of reduced clinical complexity, with significant effects in terms of

efficiency and effectiveness;

• the development of the coordination and integration allowing to better address the problems of co-morbidity;

• the opportunity to compare the knowledge and skills can improve the clinical performance;

• the long term generation of effects of scale. It is in fact possible to anticipate different services to the same patient at the same event;

• integration between general practitioners and specialists who work in the territory.

Some studies, however, indicate the possibility of **inefficiency** related to the difficulty of working together and the increasing complexity of organizational processes. In other words it is not sufficient to build formally integrated processes, but these must be built in a culture of teamwork

The centrality of the territory does not entail, moreover, only a shift of care, but also implies a change of perspective in the work of professionals who take charge not only of addressing the onset of a disease in the individual, but to develop attention in the creation of conditions that favor the development of healthy living in the community. In this perspective, the debate between **Primary Care and Primary Health Care** has a long history and has helped to develop the concept of Community Care.

With a view towards "making health burden in the community", literature indicates that primary care can play an important role in promoting health and reducing health inequalities. In addition, take care of the community logic poses the problem of **integration** between the different actors that make up the network of local services and, consequently, of governance processes to help direct the action of individual actors in the development of the territory's health and its inhabitants.

This approach is consistent with the indication of the WHO when speaking of **"health in all policies"**, as it leads to allocating to professionals working in primary care system, a central role in this process. This role allows them to activate community resources, directing them to the promotion of healthy lifestyles, and to promote policies consistent with the development of public health.

The need to move the center of the health system to the territory **confronts-bumps against the power** and the culture systems that represent the health care system in its development stage and is highlighting the strong differentiation of hospital and community contexts.

From the point of view of governance processes, **the territory and the hospital** are characterized by strongly differentiated dynamics and cultural contexts.

The **hospital** has developed following the logic of large organizations (Ford) and culture that characterized the medical knowledge, namely specialization. This structural and cultural facility has resulted in relatively closed, **hierarchical**, vertical organizational systems of power.

The turbulence dynamics regard the evolution of epidemiological patterns, clinical knowledge and technology, However, the social dynamics and the changes of preference systems of the social actors are **relatively incapable of activating change**. Its closure and stability has two implications.

The first concerns the dynamics of the actors and the distribution of power. The key players that determine the processes of government are, in fact, managers and professionals. There surely also are **dynamics of political influence**, however, these mostly concern the appointment of strategic organizations and, in addition follow informal dynamics. The ability to hack into real processes by social forces, citizens and local government is certainly lower.

The second relates to the organizational dynamics that are characterized by a **hierarchical culture** and a segmented structure because of the increasing specialization of scientific knowledge and the power dynamics between the professional groups.

	Hospital	Territory
Openness of the system	low	high
Complexity	Relatively low	Relatively high
Relation among actors	Herarachy	Net
Key actors	Manager professional clinical, (political, region)	Politicians (region and local authorities), managers, professionals, clinicians, citizens, third sector
Integration	Segmentation and specialization	Multiprofessional coordination

The **territory** therefore presents different characteristics.

First of all such systems are necessarily more open and interested in the social dynamics that characterize the individual local contexts.

The spectrum of the dynamics that trigger the **demand** is definitely wider, often linked to the presence of social disadvantage not always easy due to a clear state of disease.

This greater variability of demand is also temporal in the sense that social changes are reflected more directly in the definition of uncomfortable conditions that trigger an application for social and health interventions. The broad spectrum of activation of the demand and the frequent multidimensionality that accompanies it have as its corollary the complexity of the system, due to the presence of **different actors** who may be implicated: these actors are also not all members of the health care system but they operate autonomously in the same field of action.

Consequently, the organizational dynamics that characterize the relations between these actors are not hierarchical but recall the **network metaphor**.

High complexity, strong opening of the territorial system and network dynamics imply a different configuration of the involved actors and the power dynamics that connect them. The variability of situations, the multidimensionality of the causative factors that generate demand and the consequent lower incidence of specialized knowledge call into question the roles and power relations between the actors. As a result, the political dimension, even in its territorial dimension (local authorities), ends up taking a more important place in the strategic choices, but sometimes also in operational expenses. Outside of the hierarchical dynamics, in fact, the roles are more flexible and less structured in terms of positions of power. In addressing the issue of **governance dynamics** it is also useful to recall the dynamics that characterize the processes of differentiation and integration.

Again, the multidimensional nature of the problems requires **strong multi-professional integration** that occurs if and only if the involved actors use compatible linguistic and semantic structures and relate on the basis of a mutual legitimization. These conditions are the result of reflective processes of the construction of a senses and interpretation, based on a common reworking of the experiences.

The differentiation of contexts requires that the territorial governance processes take on specific forms and processes, capable of representing their different characteristics. In other words, health systems can not think of **colonizing the territorie**s with the same culture of government used in the management of the hospital systems. This is one of the greatest difficulties of the change process in place that should consolidate within the same system of government processes that take on different characteristics and logistics, although necessarily mutually integrated.

One of the elements of complexity of health systems is certainly due to the importance of **technology** in the organizational processes. This element is present in the hospital in a stronger way than in any other organizational system and constitutes one of the factors of turbulence and change of stimulus.

In this regard the organizational reconfiguration not only must take into account the need to align with the changing needs, but also to combine this need with the possibilities (offers) of technological change. This is meant to emphasize not only changes in health services demand, but also in the role that technology can play and is already playing. Initially, in fact, technologies were a help to the diagnostic and therapeutic process, but the web revolution has changed the scenario and today's technologies affect all the dynamics of the care process. In other words, the reflections of innovation in primary care paradigm can not be impeded from placing these innovations in the process of transformation permitted and induced by **e-health**.

Some studies have made an interesting analysis of the debate on changing the product in health care systems from application of the new e-health technologies. In their work they gave great importance to this process because they believe that the dynamics of communication, seen as a social process characterized by a major technological content, are key elements in the process of the change of health systems. According to these authors, the e-health strategies have great potential to **produce significant health effects**, but to produce real effects, it **is necessary** that:

* they be organized to maximize the **interactive communication** with users and to encourage their **active involvement** in the work care and health promotion;

* they be designed to work effectively and transparently **crossing different platforms** of communication and by connecting people and users;

* they be structured to engage people **based on their own interests** and their emotions and to meet their specific information needs.

By analyzing the effects of innovation in the dynamics of communication between those involved in primary care, it is easy to see that the **technologies are causing changes** in relation to three basic processes:

- the first concerns the construction of knowledge from a **clinical** point of view (availability of data and knowledge resulting in the rapid obsolescence of knowledge);
- the second is the integration of patient knowledge through the exchange of data or the construction of personal **databases** (even between neighboring professions);
- the third, perhaps most interesting, concerns the **change of the doctor-patient relationship** and the information imbalance of power that connects them.

This change is definitely influenced by two aspects: the possibility that every single person can make available, **through digital media**, all medical information about you; the spread of the Internet and the possibilities for exchange of information and experiences help to shape the knowledge that everyone uses in their own health management processes. Research has focused primarily on the availability of information sources on the network through which the patient builds his knowledge and establishes a relationship the doctor from a less disadvantaged position. Facing such trend, it will additionally be helpful that problem of the effects of these dynamics on health inequalities is considered. This implies investigating whether the differentiated use of internet concerning variables of class, income, level of education and occupational class end up consolidating the differences in resources (cultural than economic and social) that affect the current use of health systems.

This is an interesting and more new theme in the debate about the role of social networks in building knowledge. Absurdly we can assume that in the face of de-legitimization of the health system, the information built on the network can be held more able to influence behavior (think of the pressure groups against vaccinations, etc.). These items pose the problem of **the boundary blurred between real and believable**, and the construction of stereotypes which are (by definition) not exact.

The exchange of information and the process of building knowledge produced from **social networks** ends up playing a complementary role to the exchange of information that takes place with the medical staff. In this aspect, the Internet is an important resource in **patient empowerment** process, covering an important role in the health of the construction process.

But one can also glimpse to the other side of the coin, namely the construction effect of

beliefs based on partial or not scientifically validated information. In this case we can speak of a process of construction of shared knowledge produced by the health system. This type of knowledge is based on the diffusion of stereotypes constructed from cognitive distortions, "emotionally and not rationally shared." Social networks are a means of communication that vertically increases the speed of communication processes, regardless of the reliability of the exchanged knowledge. The research tells us that both these processes contribute to consolidating patient's knowledge and influencing the change of the relationship between doctor and patient. In both cases, in fact, **the relationship and the communication process** on which the doctor must work on, **changes**.

Professional and relationship networks , in fact, are likely to have few points of contact (in this case it would be useful to study the networks in terms of memberships, eg .: higher occupational class = more mixed networks; or are those professional networks the most mixed?). Primary care professionals can play a key role as a connector of these different networks. They are the ones which have more to do with the citizens, who are faced with their health culture and who can play (even through the processes of **empowerment**) a fundamental role in the construction of the health knowledge of patients.

Towards community care

Ultimately, the review of experiences and the ongoing debate allows individual some of the elements that can be placed at the base of the new paradigm of reference for the innovation of Community Care.

In this direction it is certainly relevant to:

- develop the sharing of **information infrastructures** that allow the networking of all stakeholders in the socio-health system;
- enable the formalization of care processes through adherence to common guidelines and Diagnostic Therapeutic Assistential Paths for **chronic diseases** with high incidence;
- identify process and outcome **indicators** that allow the measurement and verification of performance;
- implement **clinical audits**, whether individual or in group;
- implementing **training activities** and accompanying change processes for the construction of a shared working culture between different professionals and organizational units;
- clarify the **responsibilities** of the territorial level, in particular with regard to allocation of the **budget** also of group medicine, to the planning of district operations, performance and verification of the results.

Finally, the literature suggests that elements placed at the base of the new paradigm are reflected on some central processes in care work. To **focus on the patient** and build a holistic intervention process requires, in fact

- an increase of the patient's role and the development of their capacity to actively participate in managing his own health. In this perspective, **patient empowerment** becomes a central objective that guides the relationship between the provider of the care work, and those who receive the intervention;
- **to rethink the classification** of the state of health-disease. Again literature indicates that those who work with holistic logic ends up finding it difficult to classify the health of people in systems centered on symptoms, although supplemented by a record of social and environmental conditions under which such a condition develops.

These two aspects are fundamental elements to allow to create changes in the relationships between donor and beneficiary of care, but also to allow to place the relationship and the exchange of information among professionals of different bases, less dependent on the hospital specialized logic and more oriented towards the **entirety of the people**.

11. Digital technology in surgery
Alessandro Anselmo

The study of surgery through traditional texts has been revolutionized by digital technology that has enabled the creation of the **anatomy diagnosis** and **preoperative planning**.

Today, digital computer images are also able to give us the **volume** of each single organ or segments of it (such as a liver segment) with the relative afferent arterial, venous included biliary drainage.

Technology has therefore changed through the way of studying anatomy, **learning**, enabling a software contained in a tablet to display only the digestive system interactively, also allowing to highlight a single organ, canceling nearby organs, representing its relationships, bones, giving the possibility to put in transparency the single organ, turn it, display it in three dimensions.

With traditional education systems the learning curve is much slower, with new digital systems the acquisition of knowledge is much faster allowing the next generation of surgeons a **three-dimensional real view of patients during surgery**.

The visualization is possible already during the **pre-operative planning**, so as to enable the surgeon to know in advance the reports of the organs before surgery, in order to study well, for example, a tumor to be removed and the surrounding anatomical structures.

Today you can **see in advance** the resection plane with the possibility, in case for example of a liver removal, to know exactly what which are the vessels that will be encountered during the resection.

Laparoscopic surgery is a surgical technique that involves the execution of an abdominal surgery without opening the wall, consequently making a minimally invasive surgery through small incisions. It has changed the patient's recovery time by reducing the duration of hospitalization.

In complicated cases, laparoscopic surgery can be complemented by a manual device (hand-assisted laparoscopy) that helps the surgeon to bring a hand inside the abdomen, allowing total control and management of vascular structures, during the extraction of the surgical specimen. With these minimally invasive techniques, the patient may be discharged on the first day.

The minimally invasive laparoscopic surgery may be three-dimensional through the use of 3D glasses. Such **three-dimensional vision** increases the accuracy and precision through improved quality of image and perception of depth, allowing a better tactile feedback, reducing complications, hospitalization costs, better ergonomics for the surgeon and reduces stress .

When I work in a **traditional 2D surgery** I have to work to mentally rebuild in my brain through small movements, a third dimension which in fact I do not see. In three-dimensional **3D** surgery my action is much more decisive and precise.

We can imagine that between the traditional surgery and digital surgery there is the same difference that exists in seeing a film of Charlie Chaplin in black and white compared to visioning **Avatar in three dimensions.**

The digital innovations have led to the **robotic surgery** that has the same three-dimensional resolution used in laparoscopy but mainly reproduces all the articulation of the human hand through an instrument 3-4 mm of size. Within the body, this artificial hand moves in an accurate and precise way.

Still lacking the tactile feedback, the surgeon still works with the **joystick**, a manual device that needs to be practices in its amplified force.

The advantage of robotics is that the surgeon can not only be next to the patient but also at different distances: in the next-door room or even at kilometers away in **another city.**

Telesurgery is possible through a connection system, for example via satellite, but this may present several problems:

- need for stable connection
- medicolegal aspects for the absence of the surgeon at the patient' side
- high management cost
- privacy management of images
- predicting the possibility of a surgeon availability in case of emergency (eg accidental injury to an artery).

The first intervention was in **2001** with surgeons present in New York and patient located in Strasbourg. In 2004, a surgery was done by NASA in an underwater environment.

Robotic surgery is the ideal application in permitting **emergency war** relief to the battlefield and military ships through robot by securing a even civil experienced surgeon able to operate at a distance.

The simplest examples of telesurgery are represented by **telementoring** or by the presence of an expert in the operating room by telecommunication in order to tutor surgeons. The telementoring is the practice of developing driving relationships, monitoring between less and more experienced through telecommunication.

The future is going towards three-dimensional reconstruction of organs to as replacement through the creation of such **organs** with **3D printers**.

Holography is an optical technology for storage of pictorial information in the form of a very fine network of interference fringes with use of a coherent laser light, suitably projected; the image created by the interference fringes is characterized by an **illusion of three-dimensionality**.

The etymology of the term "holography" comes from the ancient greek ὅλος, holos, "whole", and γραφή, Grafe, "writing" and literally means "**to describe it**".

Israeli RealView alongside Philips has managed to complete a heart operation during which the doctors were able to view the **3D hologram of the patient's heart**[97].

As stated by Dr. Elchanan Bruckheimer who conducted the operation in 2013: "The RealView System has allowed me to work with **live hologram**: The patient's virtual heart was beating in the palm of my hand." The system allows doctors to see the heart of the patient in real time, in a hologram in the air, without having to look at a screen and without using special glasses.

Shaul Gelman, President, founder and VP of RealView Imaging also said that the holograms are interactive: you can rotate, zoom in and dissect with a pointer, being **able to see the inside**.

With the birth of the **holographic medicine**, a future mother can even meet her baby before birth.

---

97 http://www.panorama.it/scienza/salute/nuove-frontiere-nella-medicina-ologrammi-3d/ , last access 17.10. 2015

12. The new paradigm in health care: the health Commons and crowdfunding

Angelo Barbato

Crowdfunding or **collective financing**, is a collaborative process of a group of people who are using their own money in common to support the efforts of people and organizations. It is a practice of microfinance from below that mobilizes people and resources[98].

The **term** has its origin from crowdsourcing, the collective development process of a product. Crowdfunding can refer to initiatives of any kind, from the aid during humanitarian tragedies to support art and cultural heritage, from citizen journalism, to innovative entrepreneurship and scientific research. Crowdfunding is often used to promote innovation and social change, **breaking down the traditional barriers of financial investment**. In the last few years it is increasingly being invoked as a kind of panacea for all ills and a lifeline for the economies affected by the financial crisis[99].

The **web** is usually the platform that allows the meeting and collaboration of the parties involved in a crowdfunding project. According to the Framework for European Crowdfunding, "the rise of crowdfunding in the last decade comes from the proliferation and the establishment of web services and mobile applications, the conditions allowing entrepreneurs, businesses and creative people of all kinds to be able to converse with the crowd to get ideas, raise money and solicit input on the product or service that they are going to propose." [100]

Crowdfunding is an important source of funding, trigger-

98 https://it.wikipedia.org/wiki/Crowdfunding, last access 16.08.2015
99 Ilya Pozin, "Crowdfunding: Saving the U.S. Economy [Infographic], Forbes, 28 June 2012, http://www.forbes.com/sites/ilyapozin/2012/06/28/crowd-funding-saving-the-u-s-economy-infographic/, last access 16.08.2015

ing each year roughly half a million of European projects that would otherwise never receive the funds to see the light. It's **a way to give opportunities** to small entrepreneurs. In 2015 it is estimated that the funds raised reached approximately 34.4 billion dollars[101].

Thanks to crowdfunding, which finds all the elements to be able to release the most of its potential in Web 2.0, exponential increases in the near future are estimated (**millions of billions by 2020**)[102]. The crowdfunding initiatives can be divided into autonomous initiatives, developed specifically to support causes or individual projects, and crowdfunding platforms.

The one who brought the crowdfunding reputation overseas was **Barack Obama**, paying part of his campaign for the presidency with money donated by his constituents, who were the first stakeholders.

Example of crowdfunding as an autonomous initiative is the campaign "Tous Mécènes" (all patrons) of the **Louvre**. The plan was to collect 1 million euro through web community donations to buy the Renaissance masterpiece The Three Graces of Cranach from a private collector.

In Italy, the most popular crowdfunding campaign was that for the reconstruction of the **City of Science**, the scientific center of **Naples** destroyed by arson in March 2013, which has raised over one million Euros. Also interesting is the civic crowdfunding launched by the Municipality of Bologna for the restoration of the Portico of San Luca, one of the symbolic monuments of the capital of Emilia Romagna[103].

In **Italy today**, crowdfunding is **not regulated**, a minimal

100 De Buysere, K., Gajda, O., Kleverlaan, R., Marom, D. (2012) *A Framework for European Crowdfunding*, http://evpa.eu.com/wp-content/uploads/2010/11/European_Crowdfunding_Framework_Oct_2012.pdf last access 01.11. 2015

101 Sky TG24 - Economics. 16.08.2015

102 Vassallo, W. (2014) 'Crowdfunding nell'Era della Conoscenza. Chiunque può realizzare un progetto. Il futuro è oggi'. Franco Angeli, Milano, 2014, ISBN 9788891706843

but open regulation is ideal, without the need to build costly bureaucratic techno structures because it is the network that judges and awards the best behaviours.

While adhering to a crowdfunding project (new social health or artistic idea, for instance), how can one be certain of the correctness of reporting? **The value of the crowdfunding threshold** is discriminating feature because if you fail to get the required funding, you return the money to the individual lenders and you cannot launch the project. It is obviously important to demonstrate that the economic resources are effectively used for the request.

Thanks to civic crowdfunding some cities have initiated important positive practices. These include the public campaign for the construction of a **pedestrian bridge in Rotterdam in 2011**[104], the conversion of an underground storage facility in a public park in New York[105] and the one launched by the Mayor of Philadelphia in 2013, to buy school supplies[106].

Many believe that crowdfunding is a modern reworking of **historical practices dating back to the eighteenth and nineteenth century**[107]. Between the late eighteenth and early nineteenth century, the Irish writer Jonathan Swift inspired the "Irish Loan Fund", the of collective microfinance institutions fighting poverty among the Irish people. At the end of the nineteenth century the magazine The World of property of Joseph Pulitzer, launched a fund-raising from the bottom to finance the pedestal

---

103 Lorenzo Bandera, Un passo per San Luca, un passo per il welfare culturale, Percorsi di secondo welfare, 16 dicembre 2014

104 Crowdfunding Municipal Projects, a Look at the Impact of Crowdfunded Infrastructure in Rotterdam, The Cecil Group. URL consultato il 27 marzo 2014

105 Pool: A Floating Pool in the River For Everyone, Kickstarter. https://www.kickstarter.com/projects/694835844/pool-a-floating-pool-in-the-river-for-everyone last access 27.03.2014

106Mayor Nutter's crowdfunding campaign for schools raises $531k, Technically. URL, last access 27 marzo 2014

107 Calveri, C., Esposito, R. (2013), "Crowdfunding World 2013: report, analisi e trend"

and installation of the Statue of Liberty, after the Committee in charge had collected only $ 150,000 of the necessary $ 300,000 necessary.

Civic crowdfunding is one of the types of fundraising from the bottom which is enjoying greater success. A growing number of institutional bodies such as municipalities, provincial agencies, etc. Is it serving to finance public works and urban restoration activities. Civic crowdfunding advocates the overcoming of the conceptual separation between the spheres of private, public and enterprise in view of a good and a common welfare. "Civil economy is emerging, as a type of fundamentally open and social economy. It is an economy that is fusing the culture of Web 2.0 with the civic purposes. In our definition, the civic economy includes people, initiatives and behaviors that merge innovative ways to make the traditionally distinct sectors of civil society, the market and the state. Based on social values and objectives, and using of deep collaborative approaches for development, production, knowledge sharing and financing, the civic economy generates goods, public services and infrastructure in ways that neither the state nor the market economy alone were able to achieve".[108]

Equity crowdfunding is a method of financing that enables unlisted companies to raise funds from the public in respect of shares. According to the definition adopted by Consob, "we talk of" equity-based crowdfunding" when using the on-line investment to buy a real way of participation in a company, in which case, the "reward" for funding is represented by complex economic and administrative rights arising from participation in the enterprise"[109].

Typically, the submission of grant applications is done **through web platforms** that promote initiatives among its users and allow them to invest even small amounts. The activities of

---

108 "NESTA, CABE & Design Council", May2011.
109 http://www.consob.it/main/trasversale/risparmiatori/investor/crowd-funding/index.html, last access 23.03.2017

the platforms, because it addressed an audience of potential investors who are not necessarily qualified, takes on the contours of the solicitation of public savings and, therefore, is likely to be regulated. In some countries, the financial supervisory authority regulates the matter on a case by case basis, as happens for example in England in the cases of Crowdcube[110] and Seedrs platforms[111], regulated by the FCA[112].

In Italy, **Consob** issued a special regulation[113] in June 2013, enabling those who fulfil the requirements and authorization by Consob itself, to publish Equity Crowdfunding platforms. Such platforms can present to the public the capital increase offered exclusively from "innovative start-up", especially SPA (Society for actions) or limited society established by a law of 2012[114].

The **crowdfunding platforms**[115] [116]are websites that facilitate meeting the demand for loans by those who promote projects and the offer of money for users. The crowdfunding platforms can be divided into generalist, collecting projects of each area of interest, and vertical (or issues), specialized in particular sectors projects.

---

110 Crowdcube - Equity Crowdfunding, Crowdcube.com, last access 28.09. 2015.

111 Seedrs - Equity Crowdfunding, Seedrs.com, last access 28.09. 2015.

112 Financial Conduct Authority, FCA, last access 28.09. 2015.

113 CONSOB - Commissione Nazionale per le Società e la Borsa, Delibera n. 18592 -Adozione del "Regolamento sulla raccolta di capitali di rischio da parte di start-up innovative tramite portali on-line" ai sensi dell'articolo 50-quinquies e dell'articolo 100-ter del decreto legislativo 24 febbraio 1998, n. 58 e successive modificazioni

114 Presidenza della Repubblica, DECRETO-LEGGE 18 ottobre 2012, n. 179 - art. 25, Normativa

115 Castrataro, D.; Pais, I. (2013) "Analisi delle piattaforme italiane di crowdfunding". http://www.slideshare.net/crowdfuture/analisi-delle-piattaforme-di-crowdfunding-italiane-aprile-2013 consultato 28 settembre 2015

116 Ordanini, A.; Miceli, L.; Pizzetti, M.; Parasuraman, A. (2011). "Crowd-funding: Transforming customers into investors through innovative service platforms". Journal of Service Management 22 (4): 443. (disponibile anche come documento Scribd) consultato 28 settembre 2015

Through Kickstarter, the creators of the social network Diaspora have raised more than $ 200 000, starting from an initial request of US$ 10 000 in financing. The success of crowdfunding is leading not only to the emergence of a variety of platforms that act as intermediaries between those who propose projects and those who finance them, but also the opening of **new blogs and sites** that help to deliver this new type of funding.

13. Goals and indicators of Zero Disease
Angelo Barbato

The new integration of the **management** systems of the acute patient and the chronically ill need response strategies based on proactiveness and taking charge of the citizen, through prevention, care and commensurate with the level of care risk of the individual.

The development of a **"health initiative"**, i.e. a model of care that - integrating the classic "standby medicine", draws on acute illnesses - is able to take on the need for health before the onset of the disease, or before it appears or worsens, and to manage the disease itself so as to slow down the course, guarantees adequate interventions and differentiated to the patient in relation to the risk level.

Such strategies, as well as being based on the reduction of the organizational asymmetry of the standby medical model, are also funded on organizational models of **primary health care** initiatives, among which we include:

- patient-centered primary care, (**patient at the center of the system**) based the increased presence of patients in care processes, especially through information tools, access facilitation, improving quality of care (sponsored by the Commonwealth Fund and the Harvard Medical School and experimented in the British health system);

- **chronic care model,** based on the need for six key elements for an optimal management of chronic (choice of providers and lenders care, self-care support, team organization, decision support, information systems, development of the resources of the community), the presence of which, results in the effective interaction between an informed patient/ expert and a proactive team of family physicians, nurses and other professionals (designed by the MacColl Institute for Healthcare Innovation, promoted by the World health and experienced in Canada, Holland, Germany and the UK, where it was placed at the base of the new remuneration of family medicine system);

- **Expanded chronic care model**, where the clinical elements that characterize the Chronic care model are complemented by public health aspects such as attention to the collective primary prevention and the determinants of health (also promoted by the WHO and experienced in Canada).

Greater efficiency and effectiveness in chronic care management with that of enhancing primary **prevention** and combat inequalities in health; this emphasizes also the importance of co-ordination of the action taken at different levels of **socio-health system** in a warranty logic of taking charge of health needs and continuity of the diagnostic and therapeutic-care pathway.

The cornerstones of the strategy:

- response to the **urgent** need to guarantee health;

- Management and treatment of **chronic** conditions through **proactive** and structured interventions, based on shared paths that ensure continuity, efficiency and effectiveness in the use of resources for the citizen;

- Protection of **vulnerable**, not self-sufficient, low education people;

- **Promotion of health**, in terms of proper **nutrition, lifestyle** and **physical activity**.

INDICATORS
SYSTEM INDICATORS
% hospitalizations> 30 days
% re-hospitalizations between 31 and 180 days
Rate of resignation with IHC (Integrated Home Care) activation signaling service to 100,000 inhabitants
Rate of performance of HC (Home Care) per 1,000 residents over 65 years
Rate Pneumonia hospitalizations per 100,000 residents (20-74 years)

Rate of access of the residents to the emergency room (ER)

INDICATORS OF DISEASE PATHWAYS DIABETES
Process Indicators
Focus list available of pathology
% individual or group counseling (TARGET> 90%)
% patients with glycated hemoglobin in the last year
% patients with cardiovascular measuring in the past two years
% counseling (individual or group)
% of patients trained in the use of the reflectometer
Outcome Indicators
Quantity of entries in the proactive ambulatory with respect to eligible
How many drop out
Degree of patient satisfaction, by means of ad hoc questionnaire administration
% patients with Hb <7 after enlisting non-drug treatment

STROKE
Process Indicators
Focus list of pathology made available
% individual or group counseling (TARGET> 90%)
Outcome Indicators
Quantity of entries in the proactive ambulatory with respect to eligible
How many drop out
Degree of patient Satisfaction, by administering ad hoc questionnaire

HYPERTENSION
Process Indicators
Making available the list of pathology
% of individual or group counseling (TARGET> 90%)
% of hypertensive patients with at least a recording of the PA

in the last 6

Months

% of patients undergoing complete follow-up (TARGET>70%)

% patients who return to the first check (TARGET>80%)

% of patients with at least one determination of the lipid profile in the last 12 months

% of hypertensive patients with at least one CV risk assessment under the ISS

% algorithm hypertensive monitoring of serum creatinine in the last 12 months

% of hypertensive patients with at least one ECG recording during the past 12 months

Outcome Indicators

% patients with good BP control (TARGET> 60%)

Reduction in access PS / DEA

Reduction of cardiovascular morbidity episodes that required a home visit from the GP

admissions for complications Reduction IA

Quantity of patients entering the proactive ambulatory with respect to all cases eligible

Number of drop out

Degree of patient satisfaction, through the questionnaire administered ad hoc

HEART FAILURE

Process Indicators

Making available the list of pathology

% of individual or group counseling (TARGET> 90%)

Recruit at risk and heart failure patients classified by severity (prevalence failure of 1.5% with a variability of +/- 0.5%)

Patients with at least 3% of body weight recordings for 1 year (> 50% compared to the starting value or at least 70% of the load in patients in MMG)

Outcome Indicators

Reduced hospitalizations for SC and other causes compared

to the previous year

Degree of Satisfaction of the patient assessed by administering a questionnaire ad hoc

Improvement to treatment adherence and compliance

Chronic Obstructive Pulmonary disease (COPD)

Process Indicators

Making available the entire list of pathologies

% of individuals or groups counseling (TARGET> 90%)

Identification of smokers (average incidence of 26%) and workers involved in risky occupations (TARGET> 90%)

Outcome Indicators

Reduction for DRG hospitalizations due to COPD exacerbation or reduction in PS access/DEA

Reducing exacerbations that required a home visit of the GP

Therapy optimization and oxygen consumption

Decrease in the number of smokers

Quantity of those entering the proactive ambulatory with respect to the eligible

Number of drop out

Degree of Patient Satisfaction, assessed by administering a questionnaire ad hoc

14. From Rifkin's 3 paradigms to Zero Disease 3 paradigms

Bruno Corda, Angelo Barbato, Angela Meggiolaro

Man is **traveling through human history** by challenging himself to break down day after day boundaries thought impossible years ago.

During the centuries of ancient Rome and in the Middle Ages, life expectancy at birth was no more than **25 years**. In the early twentieth century, life expectancy at birth was no more than **50 years**.

In 2004 in Italy, life expectancy at birth was **79.54 years**[117].

By 2014, life expectancy at birth had reached in Japan and Italy for **82.7 years.** Currently every year a child who is born has a life expectancy at birth of **about 2 months longer** than the child was born the year before.

The Italian physicist Antonino Zichichi, believes that life expectancy is expected to reach up to 300 years[118]. According to the well-known physicist, experiments taking place in the **mega accelerator of Geneva** will allow man to have a hope of centuries-old life. Today, life expectancy, "hovers over eighty years, but it will grow exponentially. Our posterity will look to us as we look to our ancestors who had average life of 30 years." said Zichichi.

With the strengthening of **prevention** it will be possible to develop a drug so that it will always be easier to make an early diagnosis in order to take action promptly.

This push towards new, increasingly fascinating challenges must be caught in all countries of the world through the

---

117 http://www.indexmundi.com/g/g.aspx?c=it&v=30&l=it, last access 28.09. 2015

118 http://archivio.panorama.it/mytech/Zichichi-grazie-al-Cern-vivremo-fino-a-300-anni,last access 28.09. 2015

new paradigm of the health system which in addition to providing for the hospital as a place to stabilize the acute ill, would also provide the proactive land management through health initiative that will take charge of an increasingly sick elderly with a growing number of chronic diseases.

This territorial zone, according to Jeremy Rifkin paradigm can only be managed in a distributed manner with broad participation in the **commons** of all stakeholders of the territory itself: citizens' associations, municipalities, entities managers of public services (energy/ water/ electricity/ local mobility etc), reuse groups for environmental purposes of the assets, recycling-oriented waste / resource so that you throw to a circular economy to transform the rejection really resource towards a consumption-oriented reuse.

It's possible to develop complementarity between the paradigm of **Zero Zone**, based on a society at zero marginal costs, and **Zero Disease** oriented towards contrast to the disease.

ZERO ZONE	ZERO DISEASE
ENERGY	HEALTHY BEINGS
COMMUNICATION	DOCTOR/PATIENT RELATIONSHIP (role of internet in prevention and prediction)
LOGISTICS	HEALTH CARE (Management)

The concept of *'being healthy'* is based on the principle of preventing exposure to risk factors already known and avoidable, with a reasonable scientific basis of health damage, or otherwise, emphasizing the risk of exposure. Key aspects of the paradigm of health are the **physical activity** and **nutrition.**

Key aspects of the communication paradigm in zeroh disease are related to the development of the **Internet applied to health** (wearable devices for monitoring vital signs, health informatics, telemedicine, internet of things etc) that multiply the potential of **prevention and prediction** of disease.

Key aspects of the **logistics** paradigm in health care are the health management models consisting mainly of comparing the Beveridge and Bismarck models.

Even **Health Care**, like the Zone, needs to regain its engine in form of Distributed, Renewable, Circular Energy; oriented as much as possible to the reduction of the marginal costs. Health is not the monopoly of multinational bodies or regulators, but a form of energy, perhaps still in its potential form, but collective property owned by everyone. Health is not oil, is not appreciable nor negotiable, on the contrary, it has an intangible value as the energy coming from the Sun to the Earth through the electromagnetic spectrum, wind energy through wind, water and the energy of the tides.

All nations are now inevitably involved in a global process of **overcoming** the **geopolitical boundaries** of nations (zero area) and in the affirmation of the new global principles of the XXI century: the ever-increasing life expectancy, distributed energy, communication with increasingly free internet, a logistics oriented towards the sharing economy (Commons).

The spread of distributed thinking of Jeremy Rifkin applied to health until well-being, still has not found anchor on in many of the traditional geopolitical realities. This text is the contribution of the authors to the effective development of the application of the principles of the **distributed model (Commons)** applied to the fundamental service of human health and the environment. The powerful social forces that already are being developed in other sectors with the advent of a society almost zero marginal cost will be disruptive and together cathartic even in health.

We are only at the beginning, the early development of **new indicators** will have to move towards an increasingly zero disease area, zero waste, zero emissions, zero kilometers agriculture and renewable energy.